Physiological Principles in Medicine

General Editors

Dr R. N. Hardy
Physiological Laboratory, Cambridge

Professor M. Hobsley
Department of Surgical Studies, The Middlesex Hospital and
The Middlesex Hospital Medical School, London

Professor K. B. Saunders
Department of Medicine, St George's Hospital and
St George's Hospital Medical School, London

Dr J. T. Fitzsimons
Physiological Laboratory, Cambridge

Reproduction and the Fetus

Physiological Principles in Medicine

Books are published in linked pairs—the preclinical volume linked to its clinical counterpart, as follows:

Endocrine Physiology by Richard N. Hardy
Clinical Endocrinology by Peter Daggett

Digestive System Physiology by Paul A. Sanford
Disorders of the Digestive System by Michael Hobsley

Respiratory Physiology by John Widdicombe and Andrew Davies
Respiratory Disorders by Ian R. Cameron and Nigel T. Bateman

Neurophysiology by R.H.S. Carpenter
Clinical Neurology by C.D. Marsden (*in preparation*)

Reproduction and the Fetus by Alan L.R. Findlay
Gynaecology, Obstetrics and the Neonate by S.J. Steele (*in preparation*)

Reproduction and the Fetus

Alan L.R. Findlay

Lecturer in Physiology, University of Cambridge;
Fellow and Director of Studies in Medical Sciences,
Churchill College, Cambridge.

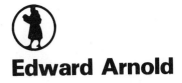

Edward Arnold

© Alan L.R. Findlay 1984

First published in Great Britain 1984
by Edward Arnold (Publishers) Ltd
41 Bedford Square
London WC1B 3DQ

Edward Arnold (Australia) Pty Ltd
80 Waverly Road
Caulfield East 3145
PO Box 234
Melbourne

Edward Arnold
300 North Charles Street,
Baltimore,
Maryland 21201,
USA

British Library Cataloguing in Publication Data
Findlay, Alan L.R.
    Reproduction and the fetus.—(Physiological
    principles in medicine, ISSN 0260-2946)
    1. Human reproduction
    I. Title   II. Series
    612′.6   QP251
    ISBN 0-7131-4442-4

Whilst the advice and information in this book is believed to be true and accurate at the date of going to press, neither the author nor the publisher can accept any legal responsibility or liability for any errors or omissions that may be made.

Filmset in Compugraphic Baskerville by
CK Typesetters Ltd., Sutton, Surrey
and printed in Great Britain by
Thomson Litho Ltd., East Kilbride

General preface to series

Student textbooks of medicine seek to present the subject of human diseases and their treatment in a manner that is not only informative, but interesting and readily assimilable. It is important, in a field where knowledge advances rapidly, that principles are emphasized rather than details, so that what is contained in the book remains valid for as long as possible.

These considerations favour an approach which concentrates on each disease as a disturbance of normal structure and function. Rational therapy follows logically from a knowledge of the disturbance, and it is in this field where some of the most rapid advances in Medicine have occurred.

A disturbance of normal structure without any disturbance of function may not be important to the patient except for cosmetic or psychological reasons. Therefore, it is disturbances in function that should be stressed. Preclinical students should aim at a comprehensive understanding of physiological principles so that when they arrive on the wards they will be able to appreciate the significance of disordered function in disease. Clinical students must be presented with descriptions of disease which stress the disturbances in normal physiological functions that are responsible for the symptoms and signs which they find in their patients. All students must be made aware of the growing points in physiology which, even though not immediately applicable to the practice of Medicine, will almost certainly become so during the course of their professional lives.

In this Series, the major physiological systems are each covered by a pair of books, one preclinical and the other clinical, in which the authors have attempted to meet the requirements discussed above. A particular feature is the provision of numerous cross-references between the two members of a pair of books to facilitate the blending of basic science and clinical expertise that is the goal of this Series. This coordination, which is initiated at the planning stage and continues throughout the writing of each pair of books, is achieved by frequent discussions between the preclinical and clinical authors concerned and between them and the editors of the Series.

RNH   KBS

MH   JTF

Preface

This book is intended to provide a basis for the study of reproductive and fetal physiology and has been written not only with the needs of preclinical medical students in mind, but also in the hope that it will prove helpful to other students of physiology and to medical graduates preparing for postgraduate examinations. It reflects my own experience in the teaching of medical students in Cambridge, in the light of which I have incorporated two particular features. The first is a thorough coverage of the post-conception aspects of reproductive function (Chapters 6 to 9) which provides the background to much clinical work in obstetrics and paediatrics, and is often tagged on to the end of many textbooks of reproductive physiology almost as an afterthought; *structural* development of the embryo is dealt with in separate embryology courses in most medical schools and is beyond the scope of this book. The second is the inclusion of a systematic treatment of the hormones involved in reproduction in the last Chapter, which is intended to supplement the attention given to the hormones in the rest of the text. Hormones are involved in the reproductive process in diverse ways, and students need to bring the strands together in a coherent account which is readily available for the non-reproductive hormones, but which tends to be scattered through several chapters in most accounts of reproduction. Reproduction is such a vast subject that omissions are inevitable. For example, contraception, and its crucial role in alleviating the problem of world population, is not covered systematically, but is dealt with in the clinical text corresponding to this (Steele: *Gynaecology, Obstetrics and the Neonate*, Chapter 15). Reproduction is a field in which studies in animals have provided much useful information, and I have aimed to cover such studies to the extent needed to place the human material in its proper scientific context.

Since the word appears in the title of this book, I should perhaps explain my spelling of 'fetus'. The Oxford English Dictionary describes it as 'etymologically preferable', and explains that the word is adopted from the Latin noun meaning 'offspring', the verb 'feto' meaning 'to breed'. There is a Latin verb 'foeteo', which means 'to have an offensive smell'; the spelling 'foetus' is therefore not merely incorrect, but might be regarded as being gratuitously insulting to the healthy fetus.

The present book was written in conjunction with the corresponding clinical text, called *Gynaecology, Obstetrics and the Neonate* by S.J. Steele, and the two books have been planned to complement each other, as have other pairs of books in the *Physiological Principles in Medicine Series*. Thus, this book does not contain a detailed consideration of the management of pregnancy, labour, and the care of the neonate; conversely the clinical book assumes a knowledge of basic physiology. Although each of these books will stand on its own, they are designed to interdigitate, and therefore each contains cross-referencing to the other. The interdependence of the two books is reinforced by the inclusion within this book of the Contents pages of the corresponding clinical text.

I was asked to write this book by the late Dick Hardy, a friend since the time we were undergraduates together. He encouraged me, and provided valuable advice and editorial comment on my early efforts. I am grateful to a number of colleagues for advice — Bob Edwards, Brian Setchell, Peter Raggett and Jimmy Steele, who has written the clinical companion volume to this text. Tony Edwards, Professor John Davis, and the General Editors have read through the entire manuscript, and Stephanie Ellington and Abigail Fowden have read several chapters; their advice was highly valued. Peter Starling and Fiona Hake helped with some of the illustrations, Jane Allsup typed many a draft, and Carol Bugg has helped in many ways. My thanks are also due to the many authors and publishers who have permitted me to use their illustrations. Judith Findlay has cohabited with this book for longer than I dare admit; to her, Matthew and Tom, my special thanks.

Cambridge, 1984   ALRF

References

Two types of references will be found in this book. First, at the end of this section, a list of General references, which are texts recommended for further general reading. Second, a list of Further reading at the ends of the other chapters. Here reference will be made to recent reviews, monographs and occasionally original papers, to which the reader may refer in order to explore more deeply the material covered in that particular chapter.

General references

Adler, N.T. (ed.) (1981). *Neuroendocrinology of Reproduction*. Plenum, New York.

Austin, C.R. and Short, R.V. (eds) (1982). *Reproduction in Mammals*, 2nd edn. Cambridge University Press, Cambridge.

Davis, J.A. and Dobbing, J. (eds) (1981). *Scientific Foundations of Paediatrics*, 2nd edn. Heinemann, London.

Edwards, R.G. (1980). *Conception in the Human Female*. Academic Press, London.

Hamilton, D. and Naftolin, F. (eds) (1981). *Basic Reproductive Medicine*. MIT Press, Cambridge, Mass.

Johnson, M.H. and Everitt, B.J. (1980). *Essential Reproduction*. Blackwell Scientific Publications, Oxford.

Page, E.W., Villee, C.A. and Villee, D.B. (1981). *Human Reproduction*, 3rd edn. W.B. Saunders, Philadelphia.

Philipp, E.E., Barnes, J. and Newton, M. (1977). *Scientific Foundations of Obstetrics and Gyaecology*, 2nd edn. Heinemann, London.

Short, R.V. (ed.) (1979). *Reproduction*. British Medical Bulletin, Vol. 35, No. 2. British Council, London.

Yen, S.S.C. and Jaffe, R.B. (1978). *Reproductive Endocrinology: Physiology, Pathophysiology, and Clinical Management*. W.B. Saunders, Philadelphia.

Contents

General preface to series   v
Preface   vi
Contents of Steele: Gynaecology, Obstetrics and the Neonate   xii

1 The development of reproductive function   1
  Sexual differentiation   1
  The genetics of sex   1
  Gonadal sex: testis or ovary?   4
  Differentiation of internal and external genitalia   6
  Differentiation of the brain   10
  Other male/female differences   12
  Puberty   12
  The signs of puberty   12
  The neuroendocrinology of puberty   14
  Further reading   18

2 The control of reproductive function   19
  External environment   19
  The neurobiology of the control of reproductive function   22
  Further reading   27

3 Female reproduction   29
  Anatomy of female reproduction   29
  The menstrual cycle   29
  The ovary   32
  Hypothalamic–pituitary–ovarian interactions in the control of the
    menstrual cycle   39
  Changes in other organs and tissues   43
  The menopause   47
  Further reading   48

4 Male reproduction   50
  The anatomy of male reproductive organs   50
  Development of the testes   50
  The adult testes   52
  The endocrine function of the testis   52

Spermatogenesis   53
Sperm maturation   57
Further reading   60

5 **Coming together**   **61**
Reproductive behaviour   61
Control of sexual behaviour   61
Coitus, and the human sexual response   62
Homosexuality   62
Transport and development of spermatozoa in the female tract 64
Capacitation   64
Activation: the acrosome reaction   65
Fertilization   65
Early development of the embryo   67
Implantation   70
Maternal recognition of the onset of pregnancy   72
Further reading   72

6 **Pregnancy**   **73**
The placenta   73
The development of the placenta   73
Placental blood supply   74
Transport of substances between maternal and fetal circulation 75
Other placental functions   82
The physiology of the pregnant mother   83
Maternal endocrinology   83
Other changes in maternal physiology   86
Immunological considerations in pregnancy and thereafter   89
Further reading   94

7 **The fetus and neonate**   **96**
Growth   96
The circulation   101
The lungs   106
Bilirubin metabolism   109
Other liver functions   110
Kidney function   111
The fetal fluids   113
Fetal and neonatal endocrinology   116
Lipid metabolism   125
Brown adipose tissue: its role in neonatal thermoregulation 125
Carbohydrate metabolism   126
The central nervous system   127
Further reading   128

8 **Parturition**   **130**
Normal parturition   130

Maternal physiology during labour   131
Fetal physiology during labour   131
Changes in tissues   132
Control of uterine activity   133
The timing of parturition   136
The dominant role of the fetus in the sheep   136
Control in the human   136
Summary   137
Further reading   137

9 **Lactation and maternal behaviour**   **139**
The growth and structure of the mammary gland   139
Lactogenesis   142
Galactopoiesis   144
Milk ejection   144
The synthesis and secretion of the components of milk   145
The composition of milk and its implications   149
Maternal consequences of lactation   151
Involution of the mammary gland   152
Maternal behaviour   153
Further reading   155

10 **The hormones of reproduction**   **156**
Hormone levels   157
Pathways of steroid biosynthesis   159
Androgens   160
Follicle-stimulating hormone (FSH)   162
Gonadotrophin-releasing hormone (GnRH)   163
Human chorionic gonadotrophin (hCG)   164
Human placental lactogen (hPL)   165
Inhibin   165
Luteinizing hormone   166
Müllerian inhibiting hormone   167
Oestrogens   167
Oxytocin   170
Progestagens   171
Prolactin (PRL)   173
Prolactin release inhibiting hormone   174
Prostaglandins (PGs)   175
Relaxin   176
Further reading   177

Index   **178**

Contents of Steele: *Gynaecology, Obstetrics and the Neonate*

While reading this book you may find it helpful to refer to the companion volume, *Gynaecology, Obstetrics and the Neonate*. The following list of contents will enable you to look up the clinical applications and relevance of the material contained in this book.

1 Normal pregnancy
2 Normal labour
3 The normal newborn
4 Resuscitation of the neonate
5 The abnormal newborn
6 The puerperium
7 Complications in the puerperium
8 Statistics in relation to obstetrics
9 Abnormal pregnancy—early problems
10 Abnormal pregnancy—later problems
11 Medical disorders and pregnancy
12 The complications of labour
13 Obstetric operations
14 The healthy woman
15 Family planning
16 Amenorrhoea, abnormal menstruation and vaginal bleeding
17 Pelvic infection and vaginal discharge
18 Gynaecological tumours and dystrophies
19 Prolapse and urinary problems
20 Sexual problems
   Appendix: gynaecological therapeutics

1

The development of reproductive function

Sexual differentiation

The genetics of sex

In the nucleus of any human cell there are 22 pairs of ordinary chromosomes ('autosomes'), and a 23rd pair of sex chromosomes which are alike in the female but unlike in the male. One of these two sets of 23 chromosomes is derived from the mother, the other set being from the father. In females the pair of sex chromosomes normally consists of two medium-length *X-chromosomes*. In males there is a single *Y-chromosome*, which is shorter, and presumably contains less genetic material than the X-chromosome with which it is paired.

Two cells contain all the genetic information that any animal inherits from its parents. They are the *gametes*, i.e. the egg or *ovum* and the *spermatozoon* (or sperm for short), and each contains 23 chromosomes. Every egg contains one X-chromosome, and every sperm contains *either* one X-chromosome *or* one Y-chromosome. The sex of the offspring of the union of an egg and a sperm will depend on whether the sperm contains an X- or a Y-chromosome. It is the presence of the Y-chromosome, and not the absence of the second X-chromosome that determines whether the embryo will develop a testis and therefore, normally, a male phenotype, i.e. a male body form.

The fertilization of an egg by a sperm results in the production of a cell (*zygote*) with a full complement of 46 chromosomes, of which two are sex chromosomes. If two X-chromosomes are present, one of them will be inactivated, but is visible in the nuclei of many of the cells of an XX individual as a dense mass of chromatin known, after its discoverer, as a 'Barr body' (Fig.1.1). Cells which may be used for observation of the Barr body include polymorphonuclear leucocytes (in which it appears as a drumstick-shaped nuclear appendage), cells in amniotic fluid of pregnant women (permitting in utero sexing of a fetus), and cells of the oral mucosa. Thus the presence of a Barr body can normally be taken to indicate the presence of two X- and no Y-chromosomes in a nucleus, but rare XXY individuals do have a Barr body.

Abnormalities of the sex chromosome: aneuploidy
If, in the course of gamete formation, chromosome division during meiosis is

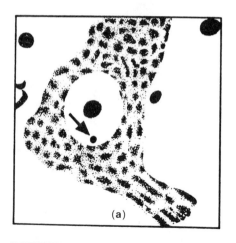

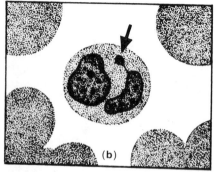

Fig. 1.1 Intranuclear sex chromatin or 'Barr body' (marked by arrow) (a) in a female nerve cell; and (b) seen as a 'drumstick' nuclear appendage in a female polymorphonuclear leucocyte. (Drawn by J.R. Fuller in Short, R.V. (1982). In: *Embryonic and Fetal Development*. Book 2 of Reproduction in Mammals, 2nd edn. Ed. by C.R. Austin and R.V. Short. Cambridge University Press, Cambridge.)

normal, we have *euploidy*; abnormal chromosomal division is called *aneuploidy*. If, as a result of maternal non-disjunction, both X-chromosomes go to the ovum then, when fertilized, the zygote will be either XXX or XXY. About one in 1000 females have two Barr bodies and are XXX (triple-X). Most are mentally normal, but some are subnormal. In paternal non-disjunction, some spermatozoa will bear both X- and Y-chromosomes, and others will have no sex chromosomes. When such sperm fertilize normal eggs, either Klinefelter's (XXY) or Turner's (XO) individuals may result. *Klinefelter's syndrome* (Fig.1.2a) affects one person in 500; they have male external genitalia, small testes, some breast development, and are normally long-legged. An individual with an X-chromosome and with no Y-chromosome (i.e. XO) will not have a Barr body; such persons suffer from *Turner's syndrome* (Fig.1.2b) and lack ovaries, are short in stature, have a female phenotype but underdeveloped primary and secondary sexual features, and have webbed skin in the neck

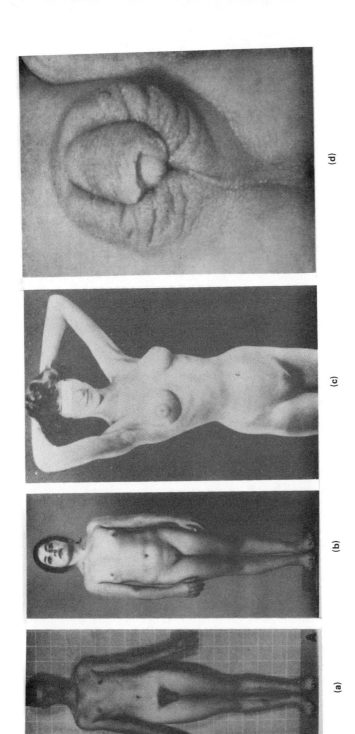

(a)   (b)   (c)   (d)

Fig. 1.2 Examples of abnormalities of sexual differentiation: (a) Klinefelter's syndrome (b) Turner's syndrome (c) testicular feminization (d) adrenogenital syndrome. For details see text. (a) From Grumbach, M.M. and Conte, F.A. (1981). In: *Textbook of Endocrinology*. Ed. by R.H. Williams. W.B. Saunders, Philadelphia. (b) From Jaffe, R.B. (1978). In: *Reproductive Endocrinology*. Ed. by S. S. C. Yen and R.B. Jaffe. W.B. Saunders, Philadelphia. (c) From Hauser, G.A. (1961). In: *Die Intersexualität*. Ed. by C. Overzier. Georg Thieme Verlag, Stuttgart. (d) From Visser, H.K.A. (1981). In: *Scientific Foundations of Paediatrics*. Ed. by J.A. Davis and J. Dobbing. Heinemann, London.)

region. Mentally their IQ is within the normal range, but they are deficient in certain abilities such as space-form perception. Turner's syndrome is seen only in three per 10000 of the human population, but more than 90 per cent of fetuses with an XO constitution die in utero.

True hermaphrodites
Most other forms of abnormality of sexual differentiation are best understood in terms of the endocrine determination of phenotypic sex, but there have been some reports of human individuals with ambiguous sexual characteristics who are composed of mixtures (or *mosaics*) of cell types some of which do, and others of which do not, have a Y-chromosome. An abnormality of early cell division could give rise to this condition. Such individuals are true hermaphrodites or *gynandromorphs*; their sexual phenotype will be determined by the hormones secreted from the gonads, and sometimes mosaics of cells are discovered within a single gonad, and ovarian and testicular tissues have developed side by side producing an *ovotestis*.

Gonadal sex: testis or ovary? (Fig.1.3)

During the first 6 weeks of development, a zygote of either XX or XY constitution develops into an embryo which is morphologically neutral, i.e. anatomically neither male nor female. This embryo will have developed a pair of indifferent gonads in the genital ridges. which are located in the dorsal body wall. These gonads have an external layer of tissue, the *germinal epithelium*, from which develop primary sex cords which come to lie in the medulla. They also possess *primordial germ cells*, which have migrated from the walls of the embryonic yolk sac and which will develop into oogonia or spermatogonia. In an embryo with XY cells, the primary sex cords in the medullary part of the gonad develop greatly, while the germinal epithelium is reduced to a thin membrane, accompanied by the production of the outermost tough *tunica albuginea*. If the cells are XX, development of the gonad into a recognizable ovary occurs much later, but eventually involves enlargement of secondary sex cords from the germinal epithelium, thus enlarging the cortex of the gonad while the medullary part regresses. After this point in the individual's development, control of sexual differentiation is delegated to hormones derived from the differentiated gonads.

How does the Y-chromosome lead to the development of a testis?
The presence of a Y-chromosome causes the development on the cell surfaces of an antigen (the *H-Y antigen*) which is implicated in testis-cord formation, though the mechanism of its action is obscure. Sex chromosomes, therefore, determine the development of the somatic cells of the genital ridge; they also play a role in determining the fate of germ cells. Primordial germ cells are present in the three-week embryo in the epithelium of the yolk sac near to the developing allantois, and thence migrate via the hind gut to the genital ridges. The subsequent fate of a germ cell depends on its environment: a germ cell lacking a Y-chromosome will normally be located in a gonad destined to become an ovary, and the germ cell will develop into an oocyte. Experimental

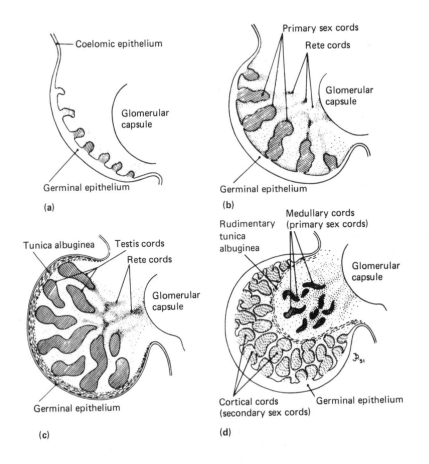

Fig. 1.3 Differentiation of the genital ridge into a gonad: (a) Origin of primary sex cords from germinal epithelium. (b) Gonad at the indifferent stage of differentiation; primary sex cords will develop further in the male but atrophy in the female. (c) Differentiation of a *testis* involves further development of primary sex cords and reduction of germinal epithelium to a thin serous membrane coupled with the development of tunica albuginea. (d) Differentiation of an ovary involves reduction of primary sex cords coupled with proliferation of cortical cords (secondary sex cords) from the germinal epithelium. (From Burns, R.K. (1955). In: *Analysis of Development*. Ed. by B.H. Willier, P.A. Weiss and V. Hamburger. W.B. Saunders, Philadelphia.)

manipulation of germ cells has demonstrated that if a germ cell lacking a Y-chromosome is placed in the environment of a testis, it will fail to develop into an oocyte. In the human, the survival of female germ cells depends on the presence of two X-chromosomes, because in XO (Turner's syndrome) individuals, primordial germ cells are largely absent by the time of birth despite their earlier normal development. Germ cells which are XY will normally be located in a testis and develop into spermatogonia.

Differentiation of internal and external genitalia (Figs 1.5 and 1.6)

The genetically determined differentiation of the testis has consequences for the development of many other tissues and organs which are dependent upon two major secretions of the testis—*testosterone* and *Müllerian-inhibiting hormone*. The latter is believed to act locally on the Müllerian (or paramesonephric) ducts to cause their regression. The former is responsible for all other aspects of male differentiation. The testosterone needed for the differentiation of male

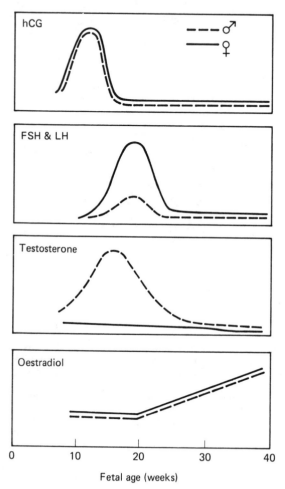

Fig. 1.4 The changing pattern of fetal serum concentrations of hormones in the human. Human chorionic gonadotrophin (hCG) rises early in fetal life in both sexes, but only the testis is able to respond by steroidogenesis early in fetal life i.e. between the 10th and 20th weeks. Pituitary gonadotrophin levels rise to a maximum at about the 20th week, and oestradiol levels rise during the second half of gestation reflecting rising oestrogen production by the feto-placental unit. (From Faiman, C., Winter, S.S. and Reyes, F.I. (1976). In: *Clinics in Obstetrics and Gynecology*, Vol 3. Ed. by D.T. Baird. W.B. Saunders, London.)

sexual structures is secreted by the Leydig cells of the fetal testis, which are developed by the end of the second month of gestation. Rising concentrations of placental *human chorionic gonadotrophin* (hCG) stimulate these cells, causing fetal testosterone levels to rise between the 10th and 18th weeks of gestation (Fig. 1.4). The rule of early sexual differentiation seems to be 'add hormone and obtain a male; add nothing and obtain a female'. Thus, in the absence of

Table 1.1 The differentiation of certain structures in the fetus in males and females. Remember that structures other than those listed may show sexual differentiation at various stages of development

Genital primordium or 'anlage'	Differentiates into:	Male-type differentiation depends upon:
Genital ridge	Testes	Y-chromosome producing H-Y cell surface antigen
	Ovaries	
Müllerian ducts	Regression	Müllerian inhibiting hormone from testes
	Oviducts, uterus, upper vagina	
Wolffian ducts	Epididymes, vasa deferentia, prostate, seminal vesicles, ureter, floor of bladder, part of urethra	Testosterone from testes
	Much regression, but part forms ureter, floor of bladder, and part of urethra	
Urogenital sinus	Prostatic urethra, penile urethra, bulbourethral (Cowper's) glands	Testosterone from testes, converted to 5α-dihydrotestosterone (DHT) in target tissue
	Lower vagina, urethra	
Genital tubercle	Glans and corpora cavernosa of penis	Testosterone from testes, converted to DHT in target tissue
	Clitoris	
Urethral folds	Shaft of penis	Testosterone from testes, converted to DHT in target tissue
	Labia minora	
Genital swelling	Scrotum	Testosterone from testes, converted to DHT in target tissue
	Labia majora	

a testis (and without the necessary presence of an ovary), the various genital primordia (see Table 1.1) show the female pattern of development. In the presence of a testis, the male pattern of differentiation occurs. In the human all the genital primordia listed in Table 1.1 differentiate in the fetus during gestation. In some species, the differentiation of these organs may be completed after birth.

The conclusions of the preceding paragraph are based on a mass of data from animal experiments, but are also borne out in studies of 'Nature's experiments' in humans. Since testosterone depends for its masculinizing action on conversion within certain target tissues to 5α-dihydrotestosterone, deficiency of the 5α-reductase that is responsible for the conversion will interfere with the normal development of those tissues. Such a condition was first discovered in the Dominican Republic. Affected individuals (known as 'guevedoces'—meaning

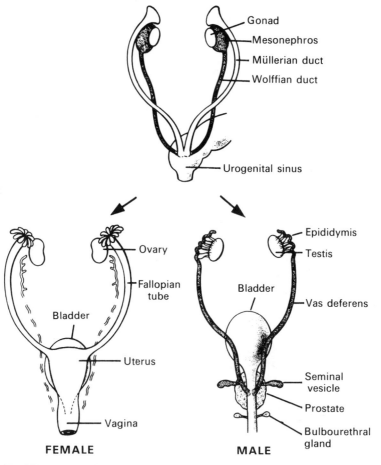

Fig. 1.5 Development of male and female internal genitalia (Adapted from Jaffe, R.B. (1978). In: *Reproductive Endocrinology*. Ed. by S.S.C. Yen and R.B. Jaffe. W.B. Saunders, Philadelphia.)

'penis at 12') tend to be raised as girls though their chromosomes resemble those of normal males. At birth they have a labia-like scrotum, a blind vaginal pouch, a clitoris-like phallus, bilateral testes, and no Müllerian ducts. At puberty, the voice deepens, a typically male body develops, the penis grows, spermatogenesis begins, and gender identity becomes masculine; the prostate remains small and beard growth is scanty. Those changes which do occur at puberty must be mediated by testosterone since the enzyme deficiency appears to persist beyond puberty.

Other individuals may have a Y-chromosome and bilateral testes producing androgens, and yet lack androgen receptors in their tissues as a result of an inherited trait. This syndrome is know as *testicular feminization* and phenotypically (i.e. according to body type) the individual is female, and frequently most attractively so (Fig.1.2c). There are female external genitalia, female body build, and breast development. Female internal genitalia are absent (because the Müllerian ducts regress in response to inhibiting hormone from the testes), testes often remain intra-abdominal, and facial, axillary, and pubic hair are absent (because growth of this hair at puberty depends on the action of androgens on androgen-receptors). These individuals see themselves unambiguously as female.

We have, then, two examples of a female pattern of differentation of genitalia

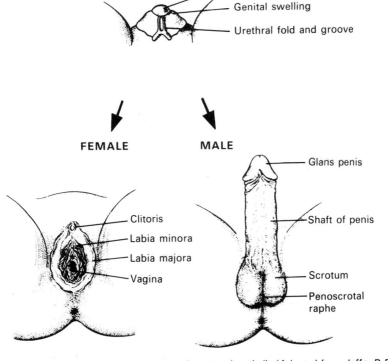

Fig. 1.6 Development of male and female external genitalia (Adapted from Jaffe, R.B. (1978). In: *Reproductive Endocrinology*. Ed. by S.S.C. Yen and R.B. Jaffe. W.B. Saunders, Philadelphia.)

when the action of androgens in genetically male human fetuses is impaired; what if female fetuses are excessively exposed to androgens? This can happen if there is excessive production of adrenal androgens by the fetus (adrenogenital syndrome) or after administration to the mother of large amounts of steroids, e.g. progestagens which produce androgenic metabolites and thereby cause 'progestagen-induced hermaphrodites'. In such cases exposure to androgens of the female fetuses is rarely enough to masculinize the internal genitalia and no Müllerian-inhibiting hormone is produced. A uterus and oviducts are present, but the external genitalia may be masculinized to a variable degree (Fig. 1.2d) and a penis and a scrotum may be developed.

In the preceding discussion, only some of the many causes of abnormal sexual differentiation have been mentioned. The aim has been to illustrate by abnormality the rules which normally operate; for a full account of the causes of abnormal sexual differentiation, the reader must seek elsewhere (see p. 18).

Differentiation of the brain

Sexual differentiation is not restricted to the genital primordia—it occurs in the brain itself. We understand this process reasonably well in the rat, but the mechanisms are less clear in the human.

The rat brain (Fig 1.7)
We shall see that an important component of the mechanism of the ovårian cycle is a surge in luteinizing hormone (LH) concentration which causes

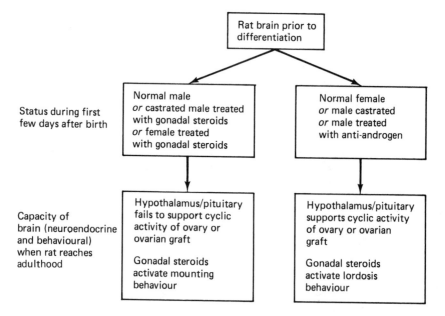

Fig. 1.7 A summary of experiments in which various procedures performed in the newborn rat can be shown to influence the capacity of the brain in adulthood to exhibit both the neuroendocrine and behavioural properties of the typical male or female.

ovulation. In species in which ovulation is not dependent on the stimulus provided by coitus, the stimulus to this LH surge is a rising secretion of ovarian oestrogens. A large rise in LH secretion follows oestradiol administration in the female rat (ovariectomized as an adult to remove endogenous oestrogens), whereas little or no response is present in males castrated when adult. This difference between male and female rats arises during the first few days of life. During this period, treatment with androgens can produce an irreversible change on the hypothalamus such that, when adult, the rat will fail to respond to an oestradiol challenge with an LH surge, and will therefore be unable to support cyclic ovarian activity. This differentiating (or "masculinizing") effect of androgens seems, oddly enough, to depend upon conversion within the brain to oestrogens, which explains why small doses of oestradiol also masculinize the neonatal rat brain. The precise nature of the change which occurs in the rat hypothalamus as a result of masculinization is not clear, but subtle differences in synaptic arrangements in the preoptic areas of male and female rats have been detected, and the preoptic area has been shown to contain a distinctive cluster of neurons (the *sexually dimorphic nucleus*) which is larger in males than in females.

Suppression of a stimulatory effect of oestradiol on LH release is one consequence of early male sexual differentiation in the rat attributable to an irreversible (*organizational*) effect of androgens on the developing brain. There is an additional consequence; when *sexual behaviour* is activated in male rats, it typically involves mounting, intromission, and ejaculation. The sexual behaviour typical of a female rat is the adoption of an immobile posture with the hind-quarters raised so as to facilitate intromission by the male; this posture is called *lordosis*. If a female rat is treated during the neonatal period with androgens, her sexual behaviour as an adult consists predominatly of mounting. On the other hand, if a male rat is castrated shortly after birth, or treated during the first few days of life with the anti-androgen *cyproterone acetate*, then the sexual behaviour of the rat, when adult, will be mainly of the female type, i.e. lordosis. These displays of male and female sexual behaviour by adult animals may be elicited either with androgens or oestrogens; it is not the nature of the hormones used to elicit the sexual behaviour which determines its pattern, but rather the brain (whether masculinized or not) upon which the hormones are exerting their *activational* effect.

The primate brain
Androgens, then, exert a masculinizing, and a defeminizing, effect on the developing rat brain. Things are less straightforward for the primate brain. Exposure of the female rhesus monkey fetus to very high levels of androgen results in masculinization of the external genitalia, and much of their subsequent pre-pubertal behaviour is more typical of males than females, e.g. more 'rough and tumble' play and more male-type mounting behaviour than normal females. As adults, however these masculinized female monkeys display menstrual cycles and if their genital development permits, may become pregnant i.e. they display female behaviour adequate to enable pregnancy to happen. Hence, in the monkey, masculinization and defeminization of behaviour need not invariably accompany one another.

The human brain

Exposure of the female human fetus to high levels of androgenic hormones can occur in adrenogenital syndrome or in progestagen-induced hermaphrodites. In both cases, there is evidence that affected (i.e. *androgenized*) individuals show some signs of masculinization of their behaviour during the prepubertal period: they tend to be 'tom-boys', and thus are more athletic and play less with dolls than other girls with whom they are compared. Furthermore these individuals have higher scores in IQ tests than unaffected girls (an unpalatable finding). However, once they pass into adulthood, they are normally heterosexual, have menstrual cycles, are attractive and attracted to the opposite sex, and can produce and rear children successfully. Humans seem particularly susceptible to social pres⸱ures, i.e. to the sex assigned to them at birth and to whether they are reared as a boy or a girl; these environmental effects will probably determine an individual's *gender identity*, i.e. subjective sense of being male or female. This is obviously a very complex issue, as evidenced by phenomena like male and female homosexuality, sex-change operations, transvestism and bisexuality.

Other male/female differences

Striking differences between males and females emerge at puberty. These include the obvious differences in secondary sexual characteristics, but there are also less obvious differences in, for example, haemoglobin concentration in blood (which is lower in women). Disease patterns differ with respect not only to the obvious, e.g. breast cancer, but also with respect to, for example, coronary thrombosis, where oestrogens appear to exert a protective role in the premenopausal woman. Culture is a powerful influence on sexual differentiation. Benign effects include matters of manners and etiquette. More seriously, the normally longer life expectancy of the female may be curtailed in societies in which governmental pressure to limit family size is accompanied by social pressure to rear a son; female babies may be allowed to die.

Puberty

The signs of puberty

The final stage of sexual differentiation comes at puberty, and involves activation of the gonads, i.e. the discharge of spermatozoa in males and of fertilizable eggs in females. Various physiological, morphological and behavioural changes occur at this time, but the clearest sign in girls is the occurrence of the first menstruation (*menarche*). Until about 20 years ago, the age of onset of puberty seemed to be falling. The average age of menarche was 15.5 years in 1900 and is now about 13.5 years. The voices of the boys in Bach's Liepzig choir in the first half of the eighteenth century broke at an average age of 18 years. This trend, which usually attributed to improvements in nutrition, general health and socioeconomic conditions, has now slowed or ceased. Chronic disease or malnutrition causes delayed puberty, whereas blind girls show slightly earlier-than-normal puberty. The age of onset of menarche in daughters correlates with that of their mothers, illustrating the importance of genetic factors in determining the timing of puberty.

The time of onset of puberty is not easy to determine with precision, but its stages in males and females have been well documented and the *sequence* in which the stages occur is similar in different individuals, even though they may take place at chronological ages differing by 4 or more years in individuals of the same sex. The state of progress of an individual through puberty can be assessed by assigning their genital or pubic hair development to a given stage according to criteria described for breasts in girls, genitalia in boys, and pubic hair in both sexes.

An obvious sign of puberty in both boys and girls is the adolescent growth spurt (Fig. 1.8), which normally occurs about 2 years earlier in girls than in

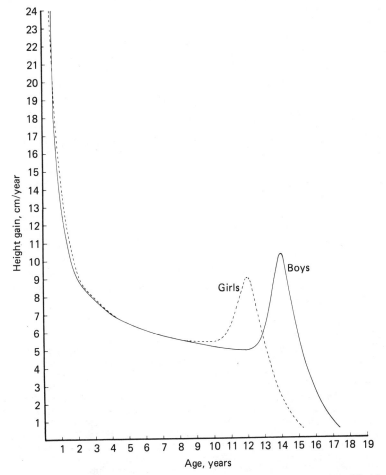

Fig. 1.8 Average speed of growth of boys and girls at different ages. (Modified from Tanner, J.M., Whitehouse, R.H. and Takaishi, M. (1966). *Archives of Diseases in Childhood* **41**, 613–635.)

boys. Thus for a short time, girls are typically taller than boys of comparable age; males continue to grow for a longer period, and thus attain greater average height. The growth spurt at puberty is caused by the synergistic actions of growth hormone and sex hormones; both oestrogens and androgens stimulate long bone growth but, later on, terminate the process by causing epiphysial fusion and the ossification of epiphysial cartilage. Not only is overall height affected at puberty, but virtually all other body dimensions. Sexual differentiation of body form occurs, with shoulder growth being greater in boys and hip growth greater in girls. Lean body mass, skeletal mass, and body fat are equal in prepubertal boys and girls; by maturity, men have about one and a half times the lean body mass and almost one and a half times the skeletal mass of women, whereas women have twice as much body fat as men. Men are typically physically stronger than women; this results from a larger size and number of muscle cells.

In males the first sign of puberty is growth of the testes and not until about a year later does penis growth or any marked development of pubic hair begin. Enlargement of the larynx, cricothyroid cartilage, and laryngeal muscles results in 'breaking' of the voice. The development of facial hair, starting with the corners of the upper lip, and ending with the sides and lower border of the chin, begins slightly later than pubic hair development.

In girls, breast development is an early sign of puberty. Then the female pubic hair development occurs, the reddish surface of the vaginal mucosa becomes dull, and the labia majora and minora enlarge. Secretion of a clear or whitish vaginal discharge precedes menarche.

Profound psychological changes take place at puberty; members of the opposite sex arouse more interest, and behaviour is modified in a variety of more-or-less desirable ways.

The neuroendocrinology of puberty

Description of endocrine changes (see Table 10.1 for normal values)
Puberty is not the first awakening of the hypothalamic-pituitary-gonadotrophin-gonadal system, but rather a continuation of development

---

Fig. 1.9 The development of the hypothalamic-pituitary-gonadotrophin-gonadal system from early in fetal life through to adulthood: (a) hCG stimulates the testis early in gestation; by 80 days, gonads are also under the influence of LH and FSH from the fetal pituitary; (b) by 100 to 150 days unrestrained GnRH secretion enhances LH, FSH, and thereby sex steroid secretion; (c) after 150 days maturation of negative sex steroid feedback and intrinsic CNS mechanisms inhibit GnRH secretion. The dial indicates the threshold of the negative feedback response of the hypothalamo-pituitary unit to sex steroids; (d) at term gonadotrophin and gonadal secretory activities are low; (e) by second week after birth gonadotrophin and sex steroids rise and then gradually fall by about six months; (f) CNS inhibition of GnRH secretion increases in infancy and threshold of response to sex steroids remains low until late prepuberty; (g) the threshold of negative sex steroid feedback rises and CNS inhibition of GnRH decreases, leading to increased pulsatile GnRH secretion; (h) adult pattern becomes established during puberty. (Modified from a drawing by Albert Miller in Grumbach, M.M. (1980). In: *Neuroendocrinology*. Ed. by D.T. Krieger and J.C. Hughes. Sinauer Associates, Sunderland, Mass.)

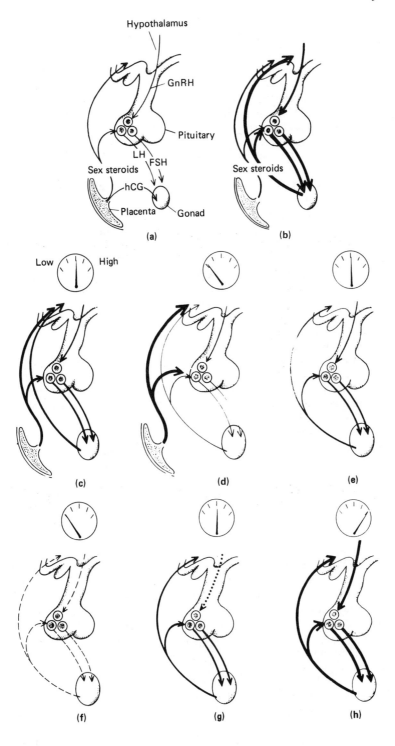

(a)

(b)

Low High

(c)

(d)

(e)

(f)

(g)

(h)

which begins in the fetus. In mid-gestation, under the influence of GnRH, LH and FSH concentrations in fetal plasma reach high levels, comparable with those in castrated adults (see Fig. 1.4). Testosterone reaches peak concentrations in fetal plasma early in gestation (about the 15th week) shortly after, and stimulated by, the peak in fetal hCG concentration achieved at about the 13th week (a in Fig. 1.9). As fetal development advances, hypothalamic GnRH secretion is increasingly restrained, and the pituitary secretes less FSH and LH (c in Fig. 1.9). This decrease in FSH and LH results from the development of negative feedback control; at birth, when the placenta—a major source of sex steroids—is removed, LH and FSH levels rise sharply (e in Fig 1.9) but will fall again during infancy. By about 2 years of age the negative feedback effect of sex steroids on gonadotrophin secretion is fully developed (f in Fig. 1.9).

The first endocrine sign of the onset of puberty is an increase in the episodic secretion of LH (g in Fig. 1.9) which occurs at first during sleep. Only late in puberty is the adult pattern of LH secretion observed, with the pulses of LH being released about every 2 hours throughout the 24-hour day (h in Fig. 1.9). In early puberty in females, FSH levels are higher than LH levels but the ratio reverses later on (see Table 10.1). In boys, plasma FSH concentrations rise progressively during puberty, whereas LH levels rise abruptly during stage 2 of pubic hair development and only slowly thereafter. Plasma prolactin rises during puberty in girls and not boys. It is presumed that GnRH secretion rises during the period around puberty, and it is thought that this is responsible for the increase in the pulsatile secretion of gonadotrophins. Gonadotrophins are released in 'circhoral' pulses occurring about every 2 hours; this episodic secretion underlies both the 'tonic' and 'basal' secretion of gonadotrophins present in males and females at all stages of life. Superimposed upon this pattern, there develops at puberty in females the 'cyclic' release of gonado-trophins which terminates with the menopause. The mechanisms underlying this cyclicity are discussed in Chapter 3. The capacity for cyclic gonadotrophin release, which is necessary for menarche, develops gradually. It depends on the development of the stimulatory, as opposed to the inhibitory, effect of sex steroids on gonadotrophin secretion. A high proportion of cycles are anovulatory during the first 2 years after menarche, but the proportion falls over the next 3 years.

Control of endocrine changes
Gonadotrophin secretion may be quite high in both the fetus and neonate but then, for a decade or so, it is in some way suppressed. One possible mechanism is a high sensitivity of the hypothalamic-pituitary system to the negative feedback effects of steroids in the prepubertal period, and that puberty is associated with a gradual decrease in this sensitivity. There is much evidence in support of this 'gonadostat' theory, but it is not the whole story because children without gonads (in whom no sex steroids would be present to exert negative feedback) show a fall in gonadotrophin secretion between 4 and 11 years of age. Thus a neural inhibitory mechanism, independent of gonadal influence, must restrain gonadotrophin synthesis and secretion, and inhibit the onset of puberty; the mechanism must be suppressed in order that

gonadotrophin secretion can be reactivated at puberty. Precocious puberty can arise when hypothalamic lesions cause premature suppression of the neural inhibition. We do not understand how the neural inhibitory mechanisms interact with the highly sensitive negative feedback mechanisms, but with the approach of puberty both neural and hormonal restraints on GnRH secretion are apparently removed, leading to priming of the gonadotroph cells of the pituitary, their increased sensitivity to GnRH, increased gonadotrophin secretion and, finally, augmented output of sex steroids from the gonads. The priming effect of GnRH is important and takes time; LH release in response to GnRH administration in prepubertal children beyond infancy is minimal, but increases strikingly around the time of puberty. While a change in the brain-pituitary axis is without doubt important in the onset of puberty, some changes in the gonads may also be necessary; gonads of animals undergoing sexual maturation show an increase in gonadotrophin binding sites, and the priming effect of FSH on the gonadal response to LH is probably crucial in this context.

Little is known of the events occurring within the brain which could explain its central role in determining the time of onset of puberty. Perhaps the onset of puberty is associated with an increase in the number of terminal arborizations of adrenergic neurons synapsing with GnRH-producing neurons. Hypothalamic control of GnRH release at puberty is obviously important, and hypothalamic lesions alter the timing of puberty. But extrahypothalamic structures may also be involved; lesions of the amygdala induce precocious puberty in rats, while chronic electrical stimulation of the amygdala delays its onset. The pineal gland has also been implicated in the regulation of puberty.

Studies on pubescent girls have indicated that a certain minimum body weight and percentage of body fat are required for the initiation of the adolescent growth spurt and menarche; the growth spurt begins at 30 kg and menarche at 48 kg body weight. The mechanism underlying this 'critical body weight' theory is obscure. Animal experiments suggest a role for pheromones from adult males in accelerating puberty in young females with which they housed. Increased daylight accelerates the onset of egg-laying (i.e. sexual maturation) in hens, and some influence of environmental lighting in the human is suggested by the fact that blind girls attain menarche about six months before sighted girls.

The endocrine events at puberty are not limited to the hypothalamus, pituitary and gonads; there is also an increase in androgen secretion from the adrenal cortex. These androgens, particularly androstenedione, contribute to circulating testosterone levels as a result of conversion in peripheral tissues, and are probably responsible for the growth of pubic and axillary hair in girls at puberty. Adrenal cortical maturation (*adrenarche*) has its onset in girls and boys about 2 years before the rise in gonadotrophin levels, but the two events do not appear to be causally linked; premature adrenal maturation is not normally associated with premature gonadal maturation. What is the mechanism of adrenarche? Adequate levels of adrenocorticotrophic hormone (ACTH) are necessary, but probably not sufficient, and increased secretion of some additional unidentified pituitary hormone ('adrenal-androgen-stimulating-hormone') may also be required. The only animal exhibiting adrenarche comparable with that seen in the human is the chimpanzee; the lack of a convenient 'animal model' has inhibited study of the phenomenon.

Further reading

Austin, C.R. and Edwards, R.G. (eds) (1981). *Mechanisms of Sex Differentiation in Animals and Man.* Academic Press, London.

Glucksmann, A. (1981). *Sexual Dimorphism in Human and Mammalian Biology and Pathology.* Academic Press, London.

Grumbach, M.M., Grave, G.D. and Mayer, F.E. (eds) (1974). *Control of the Onset of Puberty.* John Wiley, New York.

Marshall, W.A. and Tanner, J.M. (1969). Variation in the pattern of pubertal changes in girls. *Archives of Diseases in Childhood* **44**, 291-303.

Marshall, W.A. and Tanner, J.M. (1969). Variation in the pattern of pubertal changes in boys. *Archives of Diseases in Childhood* **45**, 13-23.

Money, J. and Ehrhardt, A.E. (1972). *Man and Woman, Boy and Girl.* Johns Hopkins University Press, Baltimore.

Simpson, J.L. (1976). *Disorders of Sexual Differentiation: Etiology and Clinical Delineation.* Academic Press, New York.

Tanner, J.M. (1962). *Growth at Adolescence,* 2nd edn. Blackwell Scientific, Oxford.

2

The control of reproductive function

External environment

Introduction
The control of gonadal function by the anterior pituitary gland, of the anterior pituitary gland by the hypothalamus, and of the hypothalamus by the rest of the brain and ultimately the external environment, is generally recognized. Much credit for the elucidation of the 'The Neural Control of the Pituitary Gland' must go to Geoffrey Harris whose monograph on that subject was a milestone. Since it is impossible to impose rigid controls over the external environment of man, the most convincing data are derived from animal studies; the evidence from these will be summarized for the different environmental influences and data from human studies will be mentioned where it is available.

Light
Many animals show seasonal reproductive patterns; these have evolved to ensure the birth of young at the time of year when their survival is most likely. Most start to breed as days get longer, but some (e.g. sheep and deer) show an increase of gonadal activity (both male and female) as days get shorter. When red deer were transported from the UK to New Zealand, their seasonal reproductive cycle showed a phase shift of 6 months.

Environmental lighting shows not only annual, but also 24-hour (properly called *nycthemeral*), rhythmicity. Many endocrine phenomena show an approximately 24-hour (i.e. *circadian*) *endogenous* rhythmicity which is entrained to the rhythmicity of the lighting, which constitutes the *Zeitgeber* (literally, 'time-giver). In rats kept in 12 h light/12 h dark the surge in LH concentration which causes ovulation occurs between 16.00 and 18.00 hours on the afternoon of the day before oestrus, and ovulation occurs early in the morning of the day of oestrus. In persistent light, oestrous cycles in rats cease, and they enter a state of persistent oestrus associated with ovulatory failure.

The pineal gland may be involved in mediating some, at least, of the *seasonal* effects of environmental lighting changes, while the suprachiasmatic nucleus of the hypothalamus has been implicated in the control of many *nycthemeral* endocrine rhythms.

Air hostesses working on flights involving changes in time zones have been said to show unusually irregular menstrual cycles. Blindness in girls may be associated with the early onset of puberty, while tumours of the pineal gland, which is influenced by light (see p. 24), may cause precocious puberty. Levels of FSH and LH show at most a weak nycthemeral rhythmicity in women beyond puberty but, during the period of prepubertal sexual maturation, LH levels tend to be higher during sleep, i.e. during darkness. Recently it has been shown that the ovulatory surge of LH in women (see Chapter 3) tends to occur in the morning. The time of onset of parturition shows a weak 24-hour rhythmicity in the woman.

Reproductive hormone secretion is also affected by the spatial pattern of visual stimulation. If isolated female doves are able to see themselves in a mirror, they are more likely to ovulate. In the human, few reliable data exist to link visual images to reproductive endocrine activation, though the effect of appropriate visual cues on sexual arousal, particularly in males, is well known and widely exploited.

Smell

Agents secreted into the bloodstream of an individual in minute amounts exerting controlling effects on other organs and tissues are known as *hormones*. Substances secreted by individuals of a species causing specific physiological reactions on other individuals of the same species are known as *pheromones*, and their actions are mediated by the olfactory receptors of the affected individual. Pheromonal effects on reproductive activity have been particularly well studied in mice. They include the synchronization of oestrous cycles in females housed together (the Whitten effect), the suspension of cycles if conditions are very crowded (the Lee-Boot effect), and the blocking of the implantation of an embryo if a pregnant female mouse is exposed to the smell of the urine of a male of a strain different from the one with whom she had previously mated (the Bruce effect).

There are also olfactory effects on reproductive behaviour. Oestrogens alter vaginal secretions in female monkeys and provide increased amounts of substrate for microbial metabolism; the products of this metabolism include various simple aliphatic acids (e.g. acetic, propionic and isobutyric) which act on olfactory receptors in male primates and stimulate their sexual activity. Progesterone causes the vaginal secretions of monkeys to become less sexually attractive.

Women housed together in dormitories may show synchronous menstrual cycles, possibly as a result of olfactory interaction. The olfactory sensitivity of women varies with the menstrual cycle: sensitivity to the c15 lactone 'Exaltolide' increases at the time of ovulation and is lowest at the time of menstruation. The perfume industry, which relies on animals' secretions for many of its products, would presumably be less vigorous if the human showed no arousal of sexual appetite upon appropriate olfactory stimulation.

We do not understand the mechanisms underlying these olfactory effects on reproductive function, though neural projections from structures such as the amygdala and hippocampus to the hypothalamus are presumably involved.

Touch

Activation of mechanoreceptors may elicit a variety of reproductive hormonal responses. Some mammals, including the rabbit and the cat, ovulate reflexly in response to the tactile stimulation provided by coitus; a neurally mediated increase in GnRH secretion is presumably responsible for the LH surge which causes them to ovulate. Rats ovulate spontaneously, but the stimulus of coitus elicits a sufficient release of prolactin to prolong by several days the lifespan of the corpora lutea formed after ovulation. Some have claimed that the probability of ovulation in women may be increased by coitus. Plasma testosterone levels in men are higher during and immediately after sexual intercourse than under resting conditions. The many effects of the suckling stimulus, including prolactin release, and the inhibition of gonadotrophin release, are described in Chapter 9.

When the number of eggs in the nest of many species of birds (e.g. lark, swallow and house sparrow) reaches a critical value, ovulation is inhibited, and no more eggs are laid. If eggs are removed ovulation resumes until the critical number of eggs is again reached—a 'numerical', and probably tactile, control of gonadotrophin release.

Sound

Ovarian stimulation in female birds may follow exposure to particular bird-songs. In mammals, stressful auditory stimulation will stimulate the adrenal cortex, and may inhibit ovarian activity.

Ultra-high frequency sounds emitted by baby rats may facilitate oxytocin release in their nursing mothers; oxytocin release can become conditioned to appropriate auditory stimuli, e.g. rattling milk pails in cows, or a crying baby in women.

Nutrition

Nutritional status may be determined by the external environment, but is not strictly an environmental stimulus. In animals a poor diet may delay puberty, shorten the breeding season, decrease the number of eggs shed in ovulation, and decrease fetal growth. Pregnancy and, in particular, lactation, place great energy demands on female mammals, particularly if they are small.

Undernutrition in humans may decrease fertility. Births are spaced about 4 years apart in undernourished women who breastfeed, but about 2 years apart in well-nourished breast-feeding women using no contraceptive measures. Girls suffering from anorexia nervosa typically stop ovulating and menstruating, (Steele: *Gynaecology, Obstetrics and the Neonate*, Chapter 16).

Psycho-social factors, pain and stress

Stressful stimuli generally inhibit reproductive hormone secretion. Oxytocin release is inhibited by fear or embarrassment. The stress of moving house, of anxiety, or of bereavement may inhibit ovulation and cause menstrual irregularities in women, presumably by interfering with GnRH, and therefore LH, release.

Testosterone production (as measured by rate of facial hair growth) is increased in men by anticipation of sexual activity during a period of relative deprivation. Male monkeys exposed to receptive females respond with an increase in plasma testosterone concentration. On the other hand, stress, while increasing adrenal steroid secretion, suppresses plasma testosterone levels. Males of many animal species develop a social hierarchy; the dominant male normally has the highest testosterone level, and the lowest levels of adrenal cortical hormones. In both men and women, normal sexual behaviour may be adversely affected by anxiety leading to impotence and/or frigidity.

The neurobiology of the control of reproductive function

The hypothalamus

The control of activity of the gonads involves the integration of information from various peripheral sense organs, as well as chemosensitive neurons within the brain, acting on the hypothalamic-pituitary axis to modulate the production of gonadotrophic hormones. The hypothalamus is a phylogenetically ancient component of the central nervous system and consitutes 10 g (less than 1 per cent) of the mass of the human brain. It is located at the base of the forebrain, lying above and behind the optic chiasm and, as the name implies, below the thalamus. The hypothalamus forms the lateral walls of the ventral part of the midline third ventricle, and is subdivided into a number of more or less clearly-defined areas and/or nuclei many of which play an important part in the control of reproductive functions (Fig. 2.1). These include (a) the medial preoptic area (lying anterior to the hypothalamus proper, but generally considered as part of it), the anterior hypothalamic area, and the suprachiasmatic nucleus, which together form an important cluster of anterior structures, and (b) the ventromedial and adjacent arcuate nuclei which lie just above the median eminence and adjacent to the third ventricle, and form part of the tuberal hypothalamus which is thought to contain many of the neurons which produce hypothalamic hormones. The ventromedial and arcuate nuclei form the main components of a medial hypothalamic region called the *hypophysiotrophic area* which alone (i.e. isolated from the rest of the brain) is all that is needed to maintain basal pituitary function. Many neural pathways exist within the hypothalamus to connect its various component parts. Fibres from many parts of the hypothalamus, notably the anterior areas, converge upon the hypophysiotrophic area. There are projections from medial areas to more lateral areas, which may provide the first stage in the various pathways that permit medial hypothalamic influences to be exerted on extrahypothalamic brain structures.

Hypothalamic connexions

The hypothalamus receives input from neurons at all levels of the brainstem. Though no direct input from the spinal cord has been described, release of reproduction-related hormones from both adenohypophysis and neurohypophysis is influenced by neural signals from, for example, the female

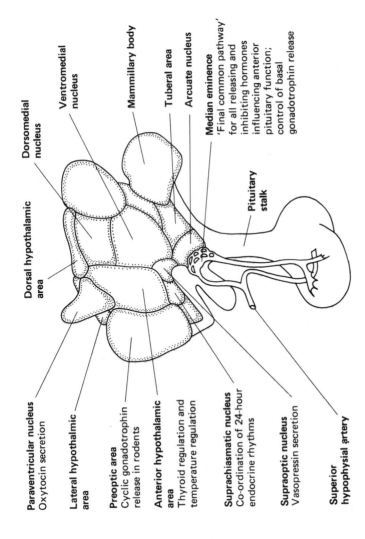

Paraventricular nucleus
Oxytocin secretion

Lateral hypothalmic area

Preoptic area
Cyclic gonadotrophin release in rodents

Anterior hypothalamic area
Thyroid regulation and temperature regulation

Suprachiasmatic nucleus
Co-ordination of 24-hour endocrine rhythms

Supraoptic nucleus
Vasopressin secretion

Superior hypophysial artery

Dorsal hypothalamic area

Dorsomedial nucleus

Ventromedial nucleus

Mammillary body

Tuberal area

Arcuate nucleus

Median eminence
'Final common pathway' for all releasing and inhibiting hormones influencing anterior pituitary function; control of basal gonadotrophin release

Pituitary stalk

Fig. 2.1 A diagram showing the various structures which make up the hypothalamus. The particular functional responsibilities of certain regions are indicated.

genital tract and mammary glands which must travel via the spinal cord. Many higher brain structures (e.g. olfactory tubercle, amygdala and hippocampus) have connexions with the hypothalamus. Direct projections from the neocortex to the hypothalamus are probably also present. Recently a direct retinohypothalamic projection has been demonstrated in a number of animals, and there is little doubt that such a projection exists in the human. Fibres arising in the retina terminate in the suprachiasmatic nucleus of the hypothalamus, and probably play a part in the entrainment of endocrine rhythms to 24-hour light rhythms.

Efferent connexions from the hypothalamus pass (1) down the brainstem, (2) to the higher parts of the brain, via, for example, the medial forebrain bundle and the mammillothalamic tract which arises from the caudal hypothalamus, and (3) to the median eminence and the neurohypophysis. Fibres to the neurohypophysis arise from cell bodies in the supraoptic and paraventricular nuclei of the hypothalamus and constitute the *magnocellular neurosecretory system*; fibres of the *parvicellular neurosecretory system* arise from cell bodies in various medial hypothalamic nuclei and terminate largely on primary portal capillaries in the median eminence (Fig. 2.2). Two products secreted by fibres of the parvicellular system—GnRH and dopamine—merit special mention because they influence reproductive functions.

Cerebrospinal fluid and the circumventricular organs

Neuron terminals do not represent the only possible source of materials secreted into the primary portal capillaries of the median eminence. Cells lining the cerebral ventricles, known as *ependymal cells*, show remarkable morphological specializations in the part of the third ventricle adjacent to the median eminence. These modified ependymal cells are known as *tanycytes*; they have numerous microvilli on their ventricular surface, and long fleshy processes which extend into the brain parenchyma, and often terminate in the median eminence adjacent to primary portal capillaries (Fig. 2.2). The tanycytes are suitably placed to take up materials from the cerebrospinal fluid in the third ventricle and transport them to the portal circulation; alternatively they might take up materials from the portal capillaries and transport them to the CSF. If the former, then it becomes important to establish the possible sources of materials which might appear in the CSF. Two sources are examples of the circumventricular organs, a series of midline structures lying adjacent to the cerebral ventricles. These organs, which include the median eminence, the pineal gland, and the *organum vasculosum of the lamina terminalis (OVLT)*, have fenestrated capillaries which are more permeable than capillaries in other brain regions, and are particularly susceptible to chemical changes in both blood and CSF.

The pineal gland arises from the caudal roof of the diencephalon and is separated from ventricular fluid by a stalk. Its only innervation is from postganglionic sympathetic axons arising from the superior cervical ganglion. Pineal function is influenced by environmental lighting and by endogenous rhythm-generating mechanisms. These mechanisms are entrained to environmental lighting by the retinohypothalamic pathway which, via several

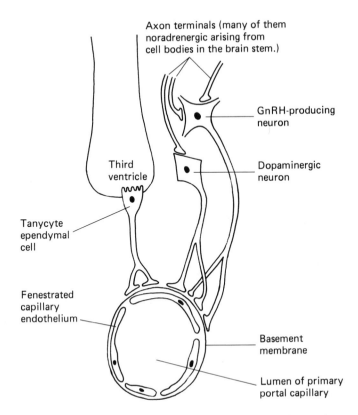

Axon terminals (many of them
noradrenergic arising from
cell bodies in the brain stem.)

GnRH-producing
neuron

Third
ventricle

Dopaminergic
neuron

Tanycyte
ependymal
cell

Fenestrated
capillary
endothelium

Basement
membrane

Lumen of primary
portal capillary

Fig. 2.2 A diagram showing three types of cell process which terminate adjacent to the wall of a primary portal capillary in the median eminence of the hypothalamus. Note (a) that dopaminergic and GnRH-releasing neurons terminate directly on the primary portal capillary, and (b) the tanycyte ependymal cell providing a potential route for transfer of agents from CSF to the primary portal capillary.

hypothalamic synapses, projects to sympathetic preganglionic neurons in the upper thoracic spinal cord. These send axons to the superior cervical ganglion—a remarkably circuitous route from eye to pineal! The metabolic activity of the pineal is maximal in the dark, and the principal product of this metabolism appears to be melatonin (5-methoxy-N-acetylserotonin). Melatonin probably has an antigonadotrophic role (indeed the various fanciful names for the pineal include 'chastity gland'). Removal of the pineal has no marked effect on reproduction in males or females of any species studied, though tumours of the pineal may be associated with either precocious or delayed puberty.

A second circumventricular organ, the OVLT, plays a part in the regulation of salt and water metabolism, but may also have a reproductive function. It has close vascular relationships with the medial preoptic area, and both structures contain GnRH-producing neurons.

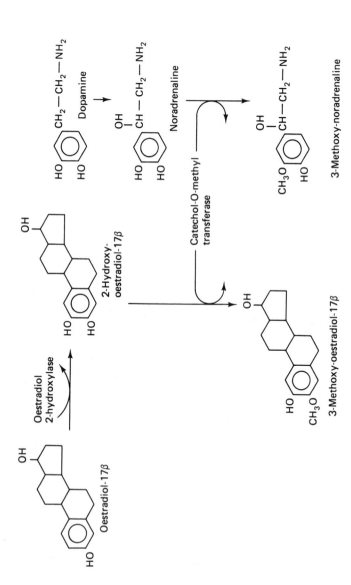

Fig. 2.3 The chemical structure and metabolic interrelationships of oestrogens (in particular oestradiol), catecholamines, and catecholoestrogens. The catecholoestrogen 2-hydroxy-oestradiol-17β has both a catechol and an oestrogen face to its structure and can react with both catecholamine-mediated and oestrogen-mediated systems in the CNS and pituitary.

The hypothalamo-hypophysial portal system

The control of the adenohypophysis by the hypothalamus is achieved via the hypothalamo-hypophyseal portal system. The conventional view of this system depicts arteries supplying the median eminence emptying into a dense network of capillaries which are heavily innervated, and which drain into the portal venous plexus: long and short portal vessels distribute blood to the adenohypophysis whence it is drained by veins which empty into the cavernous sinus. This view may need to be modified to allow for other directions of blood flow within the area, and for changes in direction of blood flow in different physiological states. It is possible that blood may sometimes flow *from* pituitary gland *to* median eminence.

Hormone binding in the brain

The reproductive functions of the hypothalamus are influenced not only by its neural connexions, but also by blood-borne agents, particularly steroid hormones. Oestrogens are bound by neurons in the periventricular area of the hypothalamus from the preoptic region to the caudal part of the arcuate nucleus, with greatest uptake in the arcuate nucleus and the anterior hypothalamic area. Outside the hypothalamus, the interstitial nucleus of the stria terminalis and the amygdaloid nucleus are amongst the areas which take up oestrogens. Oestrogen binding per cell is three times greater in the anterior pituitary than anywhere in the hypothalamus. Progesterone binds to hypothalamic neurons, but progesterone binding sites show no great specificity.

Oestrogens within the brain and pituitary gland undergo hydroxylation to form *catecholoestrogens* which may interact with both catecholamine and oestrogen receptors (Fig.2.3), causing inhibition of synthesis of dopamine or noradrenaline, or blockage of hypothalamic or pituitary oestrogen receptors.

Testosterone is also taken up by similar brain structures, though rather less avidly than oestradiol. In the newborn rat, testosterone is taken up by areas of the brain similar to those in the adult, but once there, about half of it is aromatized to oestradiol. In this site the oestradiol is believed to promote the differentiation of the male brain. Oestrogens within the bloodstream of the fetal and neonatal rat would not enter the brain, because of the presence of circulating specific oestrogen-binding protein. Testosterone does not bind to this protein and is therefore available to the brain for uptake and subsequent aromatization.

Further reading

Amoroso, E.C. and Marshall, F.H.A. (1960). External factors in sexual periodicity. In *Marshall's Physiology of Reproduction*, Volume I, Part 2, Ed. by A.S. Parkes. Longmans, London.

Harris, G.W. (1955). *Neural Control of the Pituitary Gland*. Edward Arnold, London.

Hoffman, V.C. (1973). The influence of photoperiods on reproductive functions in female mammals. In *Handbook of Physiology*, Section 7,

Volume II, Part 1, Ed. by R.O. Greep. American Physiological Society, Washington.

Jeffcoate, S.L. and Hutchinson, J.S.M. (eds) (1978). *The Endocrine Hypothalamus*. Academic Press, London.

Komisaruk, B.R., Terasawa, E. and Rodriguez-Sierra, J.F. (1981). How the brain mediates ovarian responses to environmental stimuli. In *Neuroendocrinology of Reproduction*, Ed. by N.T. Adler. Plenum Press, New York.

Krieger, D.T. and Hughes, J.C. (eds) (1980). *Neuroendocrinology*. Sinauer, Sunderland, Mass.

Merriam, G.R. and Lipsett, M.B. (eds) (1983). *Catechol Estrogens*. Raven Press, New York.

Motta, M. (ed) (1980). *Comprehensive Endocrinology: the Endocrine Function of the Brain*. Raven Press, New York.

3

Female reproduction

Introduction

The female reproductive tract undergoes cyclic changes. A pivotal event in the cycle is the discharge of the ovum from the ovary (*ovulation*). In many species, including the human, this occurs spontaneously, but in *reflex ovulators* ovulation occurs in response to the stimuli associated with coitus. Primates (including humans) exhibit periodic loss from the vagina of blood and tissue debris (*menstruation*); in species in which this occurs it is usual to talk of the female reproductive cycle as the *menstrual cycle*, because menstruation is its most evident feature. In most mammals, however, there is no menstruation, and in these the most evident feature is the periodic occurrence, at or about the time of ovulation, of behavioural change in which the female becomes receptive to sexual advances by the male, and may even actively solicit them; this behaviour is known as *oestrus*, and cycles in which it is exhibited are known as *oestrous cycles*.

Anatomy of female reproduction

The anatomy of the reproductive organs in the mature nonpregnant woman is shown in Figure 3.1. The *ovaries* are attached to the posterior body wall within the pelvic cavity. Close to them are the *oviducts (Fallopian tubes)* which communicate with the body of the uterus. There is a single uterus in primates, but most mammals have paired uterine horns which fuse at various points along their length, the point of fusion varying according to species. Separation of the human uterus into two horns sometimes occurs as a congenital abnormality. Figure 3.2 is a diagram of an ovary illustrating the various stages in the development of *follicles* and, from the remains of a follicle after ovulation, the *corpus luteum*.

The menstrual cycle

Introduction

We have seen that the maturation of the female reproductive system at menarche is not complete; many early cycles are anovulatory, and early

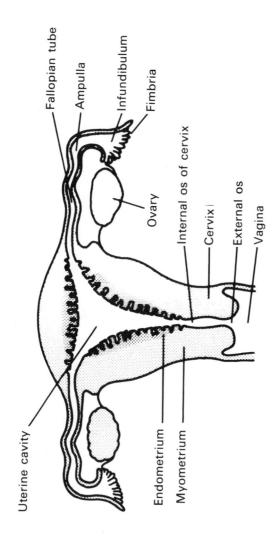

Fallopian tube

Ampulla

Infundibulum

Fimbria

Internal os of cervix

Ovary

Cervix

External os

Vagina

Uterine cavity

Endometrium

Myometrium

Fig. 3.1 Diagram of the internal structure of the genital tract of a nonpregnant woman. (Drawn by J.R. Fuller in Baker, T.G. (1982). In: *Germ Cells and Fertilization*. Book 1 of Reproduction in Mammals, 2nd edn. Ed. by C.R. Austin and R.V. Short. Cambridge University Press, Cambridge.)

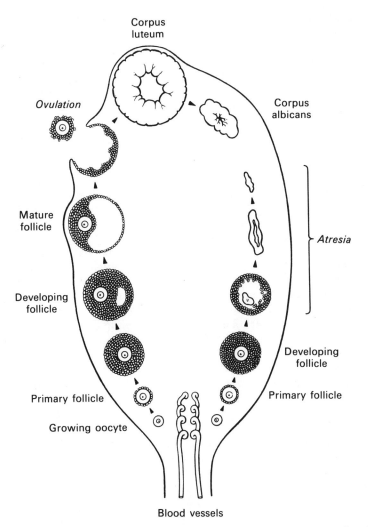

Fig. 3.2 A diagram of an ovary showing, on the left, the development of a primordial follicle to the stage of ovulation, after which a corpus luteum forms and ultimately regresses. On the right is shown the much more common occurrence of development terminated sooner or later by atresia. (Drawn by J.R. Fuller in Baker, T.G. (1982). In: *Germ Cells and Fertilization*. Book 1 of Reproduction in Mammals, 2nd edn. Ed. by C.R. Austin and R.V. Short. Cambridge University Press, Cambridge.)

ovulatory cycles are often characterized by a short luteal phase. Once established, however, menstrual cycles have a median length of 28 days. Cycles tend to be most regular in the middle of the reproductive phase of life, and are most irregular in the few years after menarche and before the menopause, the latter period being particularly associated with an increase in the menstrual interval. It has been said that 'The only regularity in the menstrual cycle is its irregularity'. In one study of a number of women, only 60 per cent of the cycles of *the most regularly cycling woman* were between 27 and 29 days in length, the range in this woman being between 21 and 33 days. Guidelines for normality are thus of necessity broad, mean and ranges being: cycle length 28 ± 7 days; duration of menstrual flow 4 ± 2 days; blood loss 40 ± 20 ml. Changes associated with the menstrual cycle take place in many different tissues and organs of the body.

The ovary

The ovary before birth

The primordial germ cells of the female migrate into the ovary from the wall of the embryonic yolk sac early in fetal life. These diploid cells, known as *oogonia*, divide mitotically between the second and seventh months of gestation. During this period they begin to enter their first meiotic division (Fig. 3.3), thereby becoming primary oocytes, and all oogonia have entered this phase by the end of the seventh month of gestation. Meiosis appears to be induced by a diffusible substance (*meiosis initiation factor*) released from cells of ovarian rete cords. This early initiation of meiotic division means that, by the end of gestation, a female fetus has all the oocytes that she will ever have. When she is born she will have about 2 000 000. The meiosis of the oocytes is arrested at an early stage, namely the *dictyotene* stage of the first meiotic prophase, also known as the *diplotene* stage; the nuclear membrane remains intact enclosing the so-called *germinal vesicle*.

The first primordial follicles are formed as early as the 20th week of fetal life as cells in the medulla of the ovary, destined to become *granulosa cells*, organize around oogonia and oocytes; this process extends outwards throughout the developing ovary. During the fifth month of fetal life, ovarian stromal tissue develops from mesenchymal cells, and some medullary primordial follicles enlarge, as granulosa cells proliferate and stromal cells differentiate into thecal cells. Some of these follicles reach the 'antral' stage by the seventh month of gestation; the number of such follicles increases in late fetal life, but all eventually will undergo degeneration (*atresia*).

Preantral follicle growth

The majority of the oocytes present at birth undergo atresia during infancy and childhood; only 40 000 oocytes, suspended in meiosis within primordial follicles, remain by the time of puberty. After puberty, a small number of these primordial follicles are recruited daily into further growth. The earliest stages of this resumption of growth involve an increase in follicular diameter attributable both to growth of the primary oocyte, associated with an increase in the synthetic activity of the cell and the laying down of cytoplasmic stores, and with mitotic proliferation of granulosa cells which secrete the glycosaminoglycans which form the *zona pellucida* surrounding the oocyte. The zona pellucida is penetrated by cytoplasmic processes, arising from both the oocyte and granulosa cells, which provide close contact between the two cell

Developmental events   **State of germ cells**

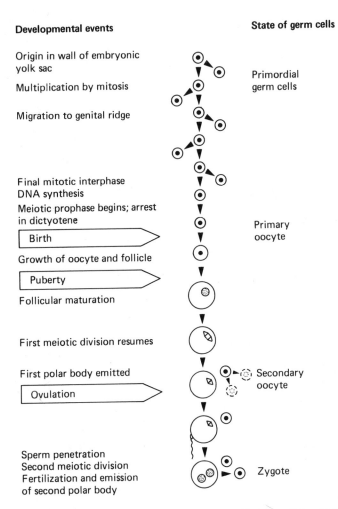

Origin in wall of embryonic
yolk sac

Multiplication by mitosis

Migration to genital ridge

Primordial
germ cells

Final mitotic interphase
DNA synthesis
Meiotic prophase begins; arrest
in dictyotene

Birth

Growth of oocyte and follicle

Puberty

Follicular maturation

Primary
oocyte

First meiotic division resumes

First polar body emitted

Ovulation

Secondary
oocyte

Sperm penetration
Second meiotic division
Fertilization and emission
of second polar body

Zygote

Fig. 3.3 Life cycle of the female germ cell. (Modified from Baker, T.G. (1982). In: *Germ Cells and Fertilization*. Book 1 of Reproduction in Mammals, 2nd edn. Ed. by C.R. Austin and R.V. Short. Cambridge University Press, Cambridge.)

types. Close contact between neighbouring granulosa cells is provided by the development of gap junctions. Flattened ovarian stromal cells surround the basement membrane (at the *basal lamina* or *membrana propria*) which itself surrounds the outermost layer of granulosa cells; the stromal cells are, in contrast to the granulosa cells, well vascularized, and become the steroidogenic *theca interna*. This layer is surrounded by a largely fibrous *theca externa*. *Primary follicles* are defined as those with a single layer of granulosa cells, and *secondary follicles* as those with more than one layer (Fig. 3.4).

Thus far, follicular development is independent of hormonal control, but towards the end of their development to the preantral stage, follicular cells

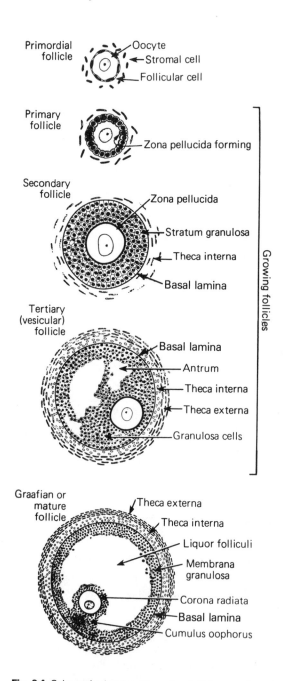

Fig. 3.4 Schematic drawing of ovarian follicles, starting with the primordial follicle and ending with mature follicles. (From Junquiera, L.C. and Carniero, J. (1980). *Basic Histology*, 3rd edn. Lange, Los Altos, California.)

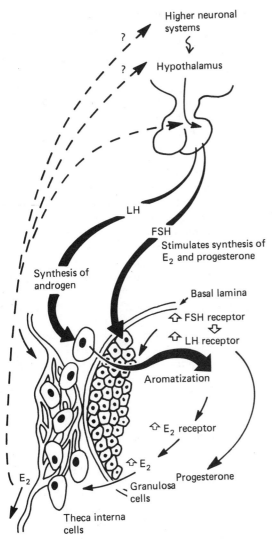

Fig. 3.5 The regulation by gonadotrophins of maturation and steroidogenesis in the ovarian follicle emphasizing the co-operation of theca and granulosa cells in oestradiol (E_2) synthesis (see text for details). (Redrawn from Yen, S.S.C. (1978). In: *Reproductive Endocrinology*. Ed. by S.S.C. Yen and R.B. Jaffe. W.B. Saunders, Philadelphia.)

develop hormonal receptors: granulosa cells develop receptors for FSH and oestrogens, and the thecal cells develop receptors for LH. The follicles need these hormones if their development is to continue.

The antral phase of follicle growth
The next stage of development, the *antral phase*, lasts between 8 and 12 days in

the normal human menstrual cycle. Many follicles reaching the late preantral stage will progress no further and will undergo atresia, in which fatty degeneration of the granulosa cells is followed by death of the oocyte, invasion of the follicle by leucocytes and macrophages, and finally the formation of scar tissue. If adequate levels of FSH and LH are present to act on the developing receptors, as they would be during the first 8–12 days of the menstrual cycle, some follicles are rescued from atresia. In such follicles further proliferation of granulosa and thecal cells can occur, and accumulation of follicular fluid results in the formation of an eccentric cavity or *antrum*. Follicles with an antrum are known as *tertiary follicles*. In a typical human menstrual cycle, some 15–20 follicles will start to form an antrum. The oocyte alters relatively little during this stage, remaining in the dictyotene stage of meiosis. It is surrounded by a mass of granulosa cells—the *cumulus oophorus*—which is connected by a thin stalk of granulosa cells to the outer layer of granulosa cells. Follicular fluid is a viscous mixture of follicular secretions and plasma transudate; ions are present in concentrations similar to those in plasma, and the fluid is also rich in mucopolysaccharides and hormones, particularly oestradiol and progesterone.

Structural changes in the follicle are accompanied by functional changes, the most important of which is the steady increase in the synthesis of androgens and oestrogens (Fig. 3.5, see also Chapter 10). The androgens — androstenedione and testosterone — are produced exclusively by theca interna cells, which have receptors only for, and are strongly stimulated by, LH. In the early antral stage thecal cells have little if any capacity for synthesizing oestrogens. Oestrogen synthesis occurs in the granulosa cells which are able to aromatize androgens, supplied by the thecal cells, to oestrogens — a process stimulated by FSH for which granulosa cells have receptors. The proliferation of granulosa cells produced by FSH has the important consequence that the number of FSH receptors increases. The follicle stimulating hormone (FSH) causes granulosa cells to acquire the aromatizing enzyme needed for oestrogen synthesis. Oestradiol can induce its own receptors on granulosa cells thereby enhancing, and acting in synergy with, the proliferative effect of FSH. This sequence of events may be regarded as a 'positive-feedback' cycle, such as is commonly found in physiological phenomena which are inherently unstable, e.g. the rising phase of the action potential, micturition and parturition. Thus granulosa cells, stimulated by FSH, respond with a further enhancement of their FSH sensitivity; by secreting more oestrogens, they enhance their gonadotrophin sensitivity still further. The important consequence is that once a follicle (the 'dominant follicle') has gained developmental headway over its neighbours, it will tend to mop up large amounts of FSH and thus its ascendancy over its neighbours will be reinforced. After some delay, exposure of granulosa cells to FSH and to oestradiol results in the acquisition of LH receptors by the outer granulosa cells, stimulation of which may be responsible for progesterone production from the follicle. Acquisition and activation of LH receptors now reverses some of the above processes; with the luteinization which follows activation of the LH receptors, receptors on granulosa cells for FSH, LH and oestradiol are decreased in number.

The preovulatory phase of follicle growth

The acquisition of LH receptors by outer granulosa cells marks the termination of the antral phase of follicular development. Many follicles reaching this stage will undergo atresia unless they are rescued by a *sharp surge* in the levels of gonadotrophin — particularly LH — which will carry the follicles into the *preovulatory phase* of their development. Normally only one follicle will reach the end of the antral phase, suitably primed with receptors enabling it to respond to a surge of LH; this number may, however, be increased in the presence of unusually high circulating gonadotrophin levels.

Shortly after the LH surge, the oocyte resumes the meiosis which it suspended tens of years earlier (in about the seventh month of fetal life) (see Fig. 3.3). The membrane enclosing the germinal vesicle breaks down, and the chromosomes pass through the remainder of the first meiotic division; the cell division which marks the end of this division is characterized by an *equal* division of the chromosomes between the two cells, but a very *unequal* distribution of the cytoplasm whereby almost all goes to the *secondary oocyte* and hardly any to the *first polar body* which will degenerate. The chromosomes within the secondary oocyte proceed with the initial steps of the second meiotic division as far as second metaphase, but then the process is again arrested. Meanwhile the cytoplasm of the oocyte undergoes changes which prepare it for fertilization. The cytoplasmic processes which provide intimate contact between the oocyte and granulosa cells are withdrawn, and *cortical vesicles,* which resemble lysosomes, come to lie just under the surface of the oocyte where they will play an important part in the *block to polyspermy* (see p. 66). These maturational changes of the oocyte are stimulated by the LH surge even though LH does not actually bind to the oocyte. Perhaps LH affects cells surrounding the oocyte and causes a decrease in the production of agents which inhibit meiosis and/or an increase in the production of agents which cause oocyte maturation.

The LH surge directly affects follicular cells causing a large increase in follicular fluid volume and blood flow. Shortly after the beginning of the LH surge there is a brief rise in the follicular output of steroids, which then falls rapidly. Outer granulosa cells from these preovulatory follicles are stimulated by their newly acquired LH receptors to synthesize not oestrogens, but progesterone, which is released from the human follicle in significant amounts several hours before ovulation.

Ovulation

As ovulation approaches the follicular fluid expands rapidly and the granulosa cell layer becomes increasingly thin, being attached to the oocyte by only a thin stalk of cells. The follicle begins to bulge out from the surface of the ovary, the follicle wall being separated from the peritoneal cavity by only a thin layer of epithelial cells. An avascular area (the *stigma*) appears in this exposed surface and the cells degenerate and the wall of the follicle bulges outward. The duration of the preovulatory phase, from the end of the antral phase to the moment of ovulation, is about 37 hours. At the moment of ovulation, the follicle ruptures at the stigma, the rupture probably arising from the activity of enzymes such as collagenase rather than from any increase in follicular fluid pressure. The outflow of fluid carries the oocyte, surrounded by a sticky mass of cumulus cells, and it is collected by the cilia of the *fimbria* of the oviduct and swept into the opening or *ostium* of the oviduct. We will follow its fate later (see p. 65).

Formation of the corpus luteum
Meanwhile, back at the ovary, the remaining granulosa cells collapse into the space left by the departed follicular contents — fluid, cumulus mass and oocyte — and a clot forms within the cavity. So begins the transformation of the collapsed follicle into a *corpus luteum*. The fibrin core formed within the granulosa cells undergoes fibrosis. The membrana propria between granulosa cells and thecal cells breaks down, and in women, if not in other species, some thecal cells become incorporated into the corpus luteum. The granulosa cells, now well vascularized, stop dividing and increase in size, their cytoplasm becoming filled with mitochondria, smooth endoplasmic reticulum, lipid droplets, a distinct multivesicular Golgi complex, and in many species an orange/yellow carotenoid pigment known as *lutein*. This *luteinization* of granulosa cells is accompanied by an increasing output of progestagens — progesterone and 17 α-hydroxyprogesterone. The maintenance of the activity of the corpus luteum in the human seems to require LH — thus this hormone is not only luteini*zing* but also luteo*trophic*. This trophic function of LH in humans may possibly be shared with prolactin, which is the major luteotrophic hormone in the rat. The secretory activity of the corpus luteum is not restricted to progestagens; in a few species, including man, oestradiol is also produced, and may well be derived from the thecal cells which are incorporated into the corpus luteum as it forms. Oestrogens may exert some control over the function of the corpus luteum; the nature of that control is unclear, and there is evidence for both luteotrophic and luteolytic effects.

Luteolysis
The destruction of the corpus luteum marks the final stage in the menstrual cycle, and normally occurs within 14 days after ovulation if conception has not occurred. The mechanism which causes luteolysis in the woman is not clear, though the luteolytic mechanism in certain animals has been the subject of intensive research which could yet hold the key to important advances in human birth control. The sheep, for example, has an ovarian cycle not unlike that found in the human; the preovulatory phase is shorter than that in the woman, but the luteal phase is of comparable length. The lifespan of the corpus luteum in sheep is prolonged if the uterus is removed. If one horn of the ewe's bicornuate uterus is removed, then the corpus luteum on the side of the remaining horn is destroyed. Thorough analysis of this phenomenon has led to the theory that the nonpregnant sheep uterus releases a *luteolytic factor* — now generally believed to be prostaglandin $F_{2\alpha}$ — which passes from the uterine venous blood into the arterial blood supplying the ipsilateral ovary, and upon reaching the ovary causes the regression of the corpus luteum; it is hard to see how the prostaglandin could pass directly across the walls of a vein and an artery, but the intimate anatomical relationship between uterine vein

and ovarian artery is emphasized by supporters of the theory. Thus in sheep, the *absence* of a conceptus in the uterus permits the release of an agent which lyses the corpus luteum; in the absence of such a destructive stimulus, the corpus luteum persists.

In contrast, the human corpus luteum seems to be equipped with what might be described as a 'built-in self-destruct mechanism' or 'planned obsolescence.' Prostaglandins probably are not involved in the destruction, though accumulation of oestrogens within the corpus luteum may be. Persistence of the human corpus luteum in the event of conception seems to arise from the overriding of its intrinsic self-destruction by a *luteotrophic* signal — namely human chorionic gonadotrophin (hCG) — arising from the developing conceptus as it implants in the endometrium. Figure 3.6 illustrates the timing of events crucial to the survival of a human corpus luteum in the event of a pregnancy.

Summary
A complete ovarian cycle is the period between successive ovulations, and lasts about 24–32 days in the woman. Prior to ovulation, oestrogens are the dominant ovarian hormones and are derived from the follicles; the preovulatory period, lasting 10–14 days, is therefore often called the *follicular phase* of the cycle. In the woman, though not in many animals, its duration coincides with that of the antral and preovulatory phases of development of the follicle or follicles which actually ovulate. After ovulation progestagens derived from the corpus luteum predominate, and we talk of this period, lasting 12–15 days, as the *luteal phase* of the cycle. The ovarian cycle described above is broadly similar in all mammals, though the duration of the various stages, and the mechanisms by which they are controlled, may differ widely between species.

Hypothalamic-pituitary ovarian interactions in the control of the menstrual cycle.

The human menstrual cycle
Accompanying the ovarian changes are changes in the level of gonadotrophins and sex steroids which are best plotted graphically (Fig. 3.7). The timing of the various peaks in hormone levels should be noted carefully; the oestradiol peak is on the day before LH surge, and there is a peak of 17α-hydroxy-progesterone which coincides with the LH surge. Ovulation occurs about 16 to 24 hours after maximum plasma LH levels are achieved. Progesterone from the corpus luteum is responsible for the rise in basal body temperature in the luteal phase of the cycle.

GnRH secreted by the hypothalamus regulates the secretion of both LH and FSH; both gonadotrophins have been shown to be present in the same cell, which supports the idea that they both *arise* from the same cell. For much of the cycle, plasma oestradiol and progesterone (and possibly also *inhibin* of follicular origin) exert a negative feedback (i.e. inhibitory) effect on the secretion of gonadotrophins from the anterior pituitary. This inhibition is probably exerted in part at hypothalamic level, decreasing GnRH release, and

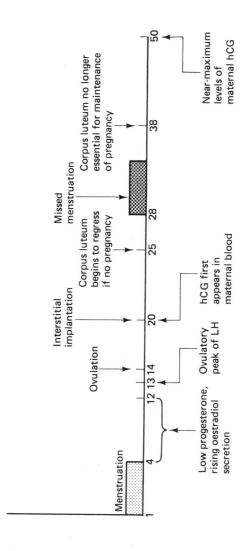

Fig. 3.6 Summary of events of early pregnancy in a woman. (Modified from Short, R.V. (1969). In: *Ciba Foundation Symposium on Foetal Autonomy.* Ed. by G.E.W. Wolstenholme and M. O'Connor. J. & A. Churchill, London.)

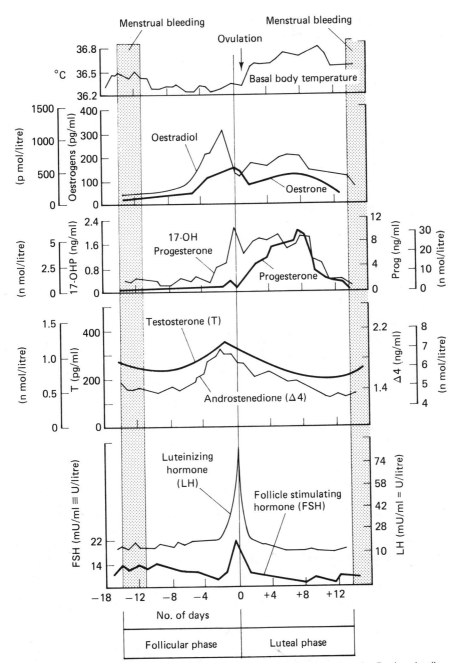

Fig. 3.7 Plasma hormone concentrations in a single human menstrual cycle. Further details of mean and range values are given in Chapter 10. In this diagram, day zero is taken to be the day of the LH surge. (Modified from Yen, S.S.C. (1980). In: *Neuroendocrinology*. Ed. by D.T. Krieger and J.C. Hughes. Sinauer Associates, Sunderland, Mass.)

in part at pituitary level, decreasing the response of the gonadotrophs to GnRH from the hypothalamus. Negative feedback is responsible for: (i) the rise in LH and FSH secretion during the early follicular phase as a response to a reduction in plasma oestradiol and progesterone levels after the corpus luteum of the previous cycle ceased to function; (ii) the fall in FSH secretion in the second half of the follicular phase in response to the rising oestradiol (and possibly 'inhibin') levels resulting from the activity of maturing follicles; (iii) the low FSH and reduced LH during the luteal phase in response to progesterone and oestradiol produced by the corpus luteum.

If the sole control of the secretion of gonadotrophins were an inhibitory influence exerted by ovarian hormones, a state of stability, i.e. a lack of cyclicity, would ensue. Cyclicity implies instability, and this is provided by the stimulatory (or so-called 'positive feedback') effect of oestradiol on LH and, to a lesser extent, FSH release (see p. 168) for a critical discussion of the use of the term 'positive feedback'). The rising oestradiol levels in the late follicular phase interact with the pituitary-priming effect of GnRH to stimulate a large increase in the secretion of LH — the acute midcycle LH surge. Oestradiol must achieve a critical level in the plasma, and must act for an adequate amount of time — at least 36 hours — before the effect is exerted. In exerting its stimulatory effect, oestradiol may again be acting both at hypothalamic and pituitary levels; in the hypothalamus, its action may well involve complex neurochemical steps including, for example, catecholamines, prostaglandins, β-endorphins and the effects of these agents on GnRH synthesizing neurons. Progesterone and 17 α-hydroxyprogesterone may contribute slightly to the stimulation of the LH surge; their stimulatory effects are, in contrast to the effects of oestradiol, exerted after only a short latent period and at relatively low plasma concentrations. Since it is the stimulatory effect of oestradiol of ovarian origin which determines the timing of the LH surge, the ovary is clearly a major determinant of the length of the follicular phase of the cycle.

We should now consider how and where the steroids exert their effects on the brain-pituitary axis. It seems clear that a major site of action is the anterior pituitary itself. When lesions are placed on the medial-basal hypothalamus of monkeys, destroying the source of most or all of the GnRH reaching the anterior pituitary, FSH and LH levels drop sharply, as one would expect. If pulsatile infusions of GnRH are then administered at a constant frequency, gonadotrophins reappear and large doses of oestradiol now cause an initial fall, but then a dramatic rise in FSH and LH secretion. This observation shows that both stimulatory and inhibitory effects of oestradiol can be exerted in the primate in the absence of any modulation of the amplitude or frequency of the pulsatile GnRH infusion; thus the steroids must be affecting the sensitivity of the pituitary gonadotrophs to GnRH. The observation does *not* show that oestradiol fails to produce a change in GnRH secretion from the hypothalamus. Does GnRH secretion from the hypothalamus change as a result of effects of steroids on the brain? A clear answer to that question is not available, because GnRH is present in peripheral blood in such tiny quantities that it cannot be assayed. It can be measured in the higher concentrations which are found in hypothalamic-pituitary portal blood — but samples of such blood cannot be obtained without substantial surgical interference, and not at all in man. It has been shown, however, that the high GnRH levels in the portal blood of the ovariectomized monkeys are reduced by administration of oestradiol — indicating that the inhibitory effects of oestradiol on GnRH release are exerted at hypothalamic level. There has been no clear demonstration of stimulation by oestradiol of GnRH release in the primate.

We are therefore uncertain about the role of the hypothalamus in the genesis of the menstrual cycle. On the one hand, the hypothalamus may be needed merely to provide an unvarying background supply of GnRH, leaving the generation of endocrine cyclicity to result from pituitary-ovarian interaction. Alternatively, there may be cyclical variations in GnRH secretion which significantly affect the cyclicity of pituitary and ovary. Whichever view should turn out to be correct, the neural control of the pituitary gland is without doubt important in female reproduction, as evidenced by (i) the disturbance of normal cyclicity by stress or by the suckling stimulus, (ii) the likelihood both that menstrual cycles are synchronized by olfactory stimuli and that the timing of ovulation is not independent of the time of day, and (iii) the crucial part played by the brain in determining the time of onset of puberty. It should be re-emphasized that the hypothalamic-pituitary system is not the only source of ovarian control: the uterus and/or the implanting conceptus also influence the corpus luteum of the ovary in a manner which varies according to species — with a luteotrophic effect of hCG predominating in the human.

Control of the ovarian cycle in rabbits and rats
In sub-primates, a role for the hypothalamus in the control of the ovarian cycle is more clear. Rabbits normally ovulate only after the stimulus of coitus. In this case a signal, presumably GnRH, *must* pass from the brain to the anterior pituitary to cause the surge of LH required for ovulation.

In the rat, ovulation does not require the stimulus of coitus, but the brain is needed to stimulate the LH surge. The surge occurs at a fixed time of day, and is abolished in female rats by: (a) lesions of the anterior hypothalamic-preoptic-suprachiasmatic region (the 'AH-SCH-POA'); (b) section of the neural projections from the AH-SCH-POA to the medial-basal hypothalamus; (c) constant light; (d) neonatal treatment with androgens; (e) treatment with a neural blocking agent (e.g. pentobarbitone) in the middle of the afternoon on the day before ovulation would have been expected.

Hence arises the concept that there exist in the rat two distinct brain sites involved in the modulation of pituitary gonadotrophin secretion: (a) the AH-SCH-POA, which shows cyclic activity (absent in male rats), is entrained to the 24-hour light rhythm, and is *stimulated* by rising levels of oestradiol thereby causing (i) a surge in GnRH secretion into the pituitary portal vessel at the appropriate time of day, *and* (ii) the behavioural changes which characterize the state of oestrus in the female rat; (b) the medial-basal hypothalamus, which is responsible for the tonic release of GnRH, and is the site at which oestradiol acts in the brain to inhibit GnRH release.

Changes in other organs and tissues

As a result of the changing levels of ovarian hormones during the menstrual cycle, there are alterations in the structure and function of various target organs. The hypothalamus and the anterior pituitary gland have already been mentioned, but what of other parts of the body?

The endometrium (Fig. 3.8)
Changes in the endometrium — the inner lining of the uterus — during the cycle reflect its different roles in the woman's reproductive life. During the follicular phase it provides a suitable environment for spermatozoa *en route* from the cervix to the oviducts. In the luteal phase it contributes to the removal of the zona pellucida from the fertilized ovum and the nutrition of the blastocyst, and later it provides a site suitable for the attachment and implantation of the blastocyst. During menstruation, the endometrial lining built up during the previous cycle undergoes desquamation. This process is associated with the disintegration of endometrial stromal cells and the occurrence of diffuse interstitial haemorrhages in the upper two-thirds of the endometrium. Leucocytes invade the tissue and separate the endometrial glands. Desquamation can continue into the third day after the onset of menstrual bleeding, but regenerative changes involving regrowth of epithelium begin on the previous day and last until the fifth day. Regeneration does not involve stromal cells, and occurs when circulating steroid levels are low. It is considered to be a direct response to tissue loss, rather than to hormone influence.

After menstruation ceases, the endometrium is just 1–2 mm thick. Cuboidal cells line both the surface and the collapsed, narrow endometrial glands. During the *proliferative phase* of the cycle, which corresponds with the follicular phase of the ovarian cycle, there occurs, under the influence of oestrogens, marked proliferation of epithelial and stromal cells — mitotic figures being abundant in both cell types. The endometrial glands become longer, and their lining cells assume a pseudostratified appearance. The cells lining the surface epithelium become columnar. During the proliferative phase, oestrogens act by binding to the oestrogen receptors which are abundant in uterine tissue. One of their most important actions is the induction of intracellular progesterone receptors, thereby preparing the tissue to respond to the rising progesterone levels in the luteal phase of the ovarian

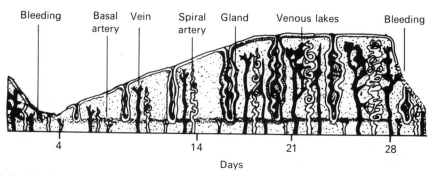

Fig. 3.8 Morphological changes in the uterine mucosa during the menstrual cycle. (From Odell, W.D. and Moyer, D.L. (1971). *Physiology of Reproduction*. C.V. Mosby, St Louis.)

cycle thus producing the changes characteristic of the *secretory phase* of the endometrial cycle. The first histological sign of the action of progesterone is the appearance, 2 days after ovulation, of glycogen-rich vacuoles in the gland cells. Blood vessels become prominent and the glands increasingly tortuous. Glandular secretion is profuse, and the endometrial stroma becomes oedematous. The thickness of the endometrium increases to about 6 mm, and in the middle of the secretory phase (and only during that period) the endometrium is ready for implantation. At the end of the secretory phase, assuming implantation of an embryo has not occurred, signs of glandular exhaustion appear. The glands begin to collapse and fragment, and leucocytic invasion heralds the onset of autolytic changes which result in *menstruation*.

Menstruation is associated with ischaemia of the endometrium followed by dilatation of the coiled arteries which supply it. It occurs after normal ovulatory cycles, but may also be seen during anovulatory states, and following the administration of natural and synthetic oestrogens and progestagens. The precise causal factors are not known, but probably involve withdrawal of oestrogens and progestagens, and the build up of prostaglandins. $PGF_{2\alpha}$, a potent vasoconstrictor, may well be involved in producing the initial endometrial ischaemia by causing constriction of the spiral arteries.

The myometrium

The myometrium undergoes low frequency (about 30/h) high amplitude contractions during menstruation, which give way to more frequent contractions (80/h) by day 6 of the cycle. At the time of ovulation high frequency (200/h) low amplitude contractions are observed, and the frequency of contraction falls to about 80/h at low amplitude by day 26. As menstruation approaches, the frequency of contractions continues to decrease while the amplitude rises rapidly. The pattern of contractile activity presumably results from the combined effects of oestrogens, progestagens, and prostaglandins (see Chapter 10).

The oviduct

The oviduct (or Fallopian tube) is a thin muscular tube lined with a ciliated secretory columnar epithelium. Fertilization occurs within the oviduct when spermatozoa, passing up from the isthmic junction, meet the ovum coming down from the fimbriated ostium. The oviduct is thus the site for transport for both male and female gametes, for fertilization, and for the initial stages of embryonic life.

Rising oestrogen levels in the follicular phase of the cycle enhance the development of cilia in the oviducts, increase secretory activity, and enhance muscle contractions. During the luteal phase, under the influence of progesterone, the cilia decline in number, secretion is reduced and the oviductal muscle relaxes — notably at the utero-tubal junction.

The cervix

The cervix lies on the route taken by spermatozoa after coitus; its properties change markedly during the menstrual cycle. In the follicular phase, under the influence of oestrogens, it becomes more vascular and oedematous, the smooth muscle relaxes and the epithelium becomes more secretory. In the luteal phase secretion is reduced and the cervix is firmer. The effect of these changes is to alter the penetrability of the cervix by spermatozoa, which is maximal at the time of ovulation, and low during the luteal phase (see p. 64).

The vagina
In the vagina of many species including the human, and most notably in the rat, there is an increase in the mitotic activity of vaginal epithelial cells during the follicular phase as a result of rising oestrogen levels. The epithelium tends to keratinize. Alterations also occur in vaginal *secretions* in association with the menstrual cycle, with consequent changes in the production of aliphatic acids by vaginal bacteria, which cause the female — particularly the female monkey — to become attractive to males at physiologically appropriate times in the menstrual cycle.

Miscellaneous effects
There are changes in the breast associated with the menstrual cycle. These are described in Chapter 9. There are also changes in body electrolyte balance: the activity of the renin-angiotensin-aldosterone system alters, causing retention of sodium and water during the luteal phase of the cycle.

The brain and behaviour
The brain is a target site for the action of sex steroids, and its activity alters with the menstrual cycle. The endocrine activity of the hypothalamus has been discussed, but what of other brain functions? The hypothalamic set-point for body temperature regulation rises shortly after ovulation as a result of rising progesterone levels. There is also, in some women, a change of mood during the days preceding menstruation. A state of *premenstrual tension* (PMT) is now well recognized (Steele: *Gynaecology, Obstetrics and the Neonate,* Chapter 16). Women, when suffering from PMT, become more liable to suffer from migraines, break the law, be admitted to psychiatric hospitals, and attempt suicide. Premenstrual tension frequently coincides with the period when fluid retention is high, and a causal link between the somatic and the physiological signs and symptoms has been suggested.

The most striking effect of the ovarian cycle on the brain function in many mammals is on sexual receptivity. Females of many species will permit copulation by the male only when they are in a behavioural state of *oestrus* (a word derived from the Greek word for the gad-fly or bot-fly of the genus *Oestridae* which cause cattle to become frenzied when they approach). Oestrus is restricted to that period of the cycle during which copulation will be most likely to result in fertilization. In animals such as the cat which ovulate as a reflex response to copulation, the oestrus state continues until copulation occurs.

In some primate species, there are cyclical variations in the sexual activity of male–female pairs; these depend on variations in the attractiveness of the female to the male, which are due to changes in the odours emitted from the vagina. The odours are most attractive when oestrogen levels are high, and become less attractive as progesterone levels rise in the luteal phase of the cycle.

In the human, cyclical variation in sexual behaviour is less clear. Sexual activity decreases during menstruation itself, and couples may also show a slight reduction in the frequency of sexual interaction about midway through the luteal phase of the cycle; this may be due to a reduction in the initiation of sexual interaction by the man, perhaps because the woman may be less attractive to the man at this stage of the cycle as a result of subtle changes in olfactory communication. Clinical data indicate that oestrogens are not in themselves responsible for 'libido' in the human, but women lacking oestrogens fail to produce the secretions which normally lubricate the vagina and experience discomfort during sexual intercourse (*dyspareunia*). Female libido in primates may be stimulated by androgens secreted by the adrenal cortex; there are experiments to back this view in monkeys, though evidence in the human is based only on clinical anecdote, e.g. women taking the anti-androgen, cyproterone acetate, frequently notice reduced libido.

The menopause

The menopause occurs between 45 and 55 years of age, and is usually preceded by increasing length and irregularity of menstrual cycles, and a decrease in menstrual flow (Steele: *Gynaecology, Obstetrics and the Neonate,* Chapter 14). During the period leading up to the menopause the number of follicles in the ovaries will have fallen to about 10 000, but the responsiveness of the remaining follicles to gonadotrophins is greatly reduced. They secrete less oestradiol, and gradually fail to ovulate. The resulting period of reduced fertility and ovarian activity, which may last for 10 years or more, is known as the *climacteric,* and during it menstrual flow ceases (the menopause), and there are also somatic changes resulting from oestrogen deficiency. The menopause is a consequence of *ovarian* failure. (Puberty is, by contrast, the result of maturational changes within the CNS.) This ovarian failure, resulting from an exhaustion of ovarian germ cells, normally occurs after the age of 40 years, but can occur much earlier in cases of 'premature menopause'.

After the menopause, oestradiol and progeterone levels fall and this results in a progressive rise in FSH and LH secretion (Fig. 3.9). Sex steroids are not absent in the postmenopausal woman, but her major site of origin is the adrenal cortex. Although the ovaries largely cease to produce oestrogens and progesterone, they do secrete testosterone, dehydroepiandrosterone and 17α-hydroxyprogesterone. Peripheral conversion in adipose tissue of androgens to oestrogens may explain the persistence of oestrogens in post-menopausal women at levels adequate to prevent symptoms of deficiency.

The climacteric may be associated with vasomotor and/or autonomic disturbance causing 'hot flushes' and 'night sweats'. The risk of coronary thrombosis rises in postmenopausal women. Bone demineralization, causing osteoporosis and increased liability to bone fractures, occurs after the menopause; oestrogen therapy retards this process. The target organs for the female reproductive steroids — uterus, oviducts, cervix and breasts — undergo atrophy after the menopause. Vaginal epithelium atrophies and vaginal secretions become scant and more alkaline. The vaginal dryness can cause dyspareunia, and the vaginal wall becomes more prone to laceration and

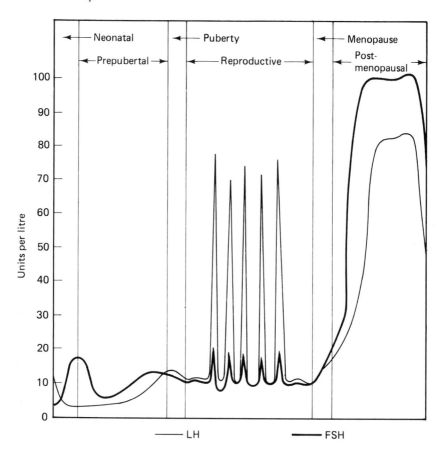

Fig. 3.9 The pattern of gonadotrophin secretion during the lifetime of a human female showing the major shifts in plasma concentration. No attempt is made to depict short-term fluctuations, nor to represent all the cyclic changes during the reproductive period. Details of mean and range values are given in Table 10.1. (Modified from Yen, S.S.C. (1980). In: *Neuroendocrinology*. Ed. by D.T. Krieger and J.C. Hughes. Sinauer Associates, Sunderland, Mass.)

infection. Behavioural disorders are quite common during the climacteric, and may include depression and anxiety. There may also be loss of libido. There is no simple connexion between these behavioural problems and the changing hormonal levels.

Further reading

Beard, R.J. (ed)(1976). *The Menopause*. MTP, Lancaster.
Crighton, D.B., Haynes, N.B., Foxcroft, G.R. and Lamming, G.E. (eds)(1978). *Control of Ovulation*. Butterworths, London.
Crosignani, P.G. and Mishell, D.R. (eds)(1976). *Ovulation in the Human*. Academic Press, London.

Finn, C.A. and Porter, D.G. (1975). *The Uterus.* Elek Science, London.
Friedman, R.C. (ed)(1982). *Behavior and the Menstrual Cycle.* Marcel Dekker, Basel. .
Greenwald, G.S. and Terranova, P.F. (eds)(1983). *Factors Regulating Ovarian Function.* Raven Press, New York.
Johnson, A.D. and Foley, C.W. (eds)(1974). *The Oviduct and its Functions.* Academic Press, New York.
Pauerstein, C.J. (1974). *The Fallopian Tube: A Reappraisal.* Lea and Febiger, Philadelphia.
Peters, H. and McNatty, K.P. (1980). *The Ovary: a Correlation of Structure and Function in Mammals.* Granada, London.
Zuckerman, Lord and Wier, B.J. (eds)(1977). *The Ovary,* 2nd edn. Vols I, II and III. Academic Press, New York.

4

Male reproduction

The anatomy of male reproductive organs

Figures 4.1 and 4.2 provide as much information as will be needed to make sense of the following account of male reproductive physiology.

Development of the testes

The presence of a Y-chromosome leads to the formation of a pair of fetal testes from undifferentiated genital ridges; the secretions of these testes are crucial to the establishment of the male phenotype. The testis first develops from the genital ridge in the upper lumbar region of the fetus. In the female the ovaries retain this position throughout life, whereas in the male the testes migrate

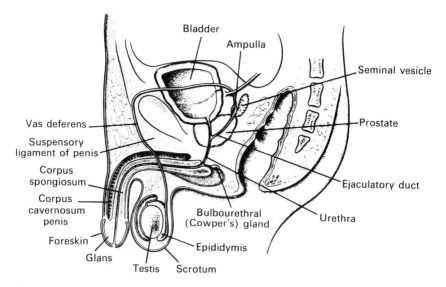

Fig. 4.1 Lower part of the trunk in a man, showing the reproductive tract and neighbouring organs. (Drawn by J.R. Fuller from M.J.K. Harper (1982). In: *Germ Cells and Fertilization*. Book 1 of Reproduction in Mammals, 2nd edn. Ed. by C.R. Austin and R.V. Short. Cambridge University Press, Cambridge.)

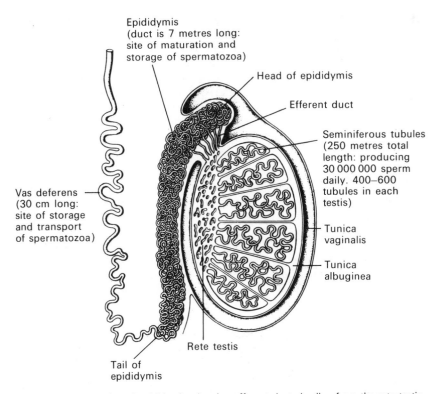

Fig. 4.2 Human testis and epididymis, showing efferent ducts leading from the rete testis to the head (caput) of the epididymis and the tail (cauda) of the epididymis continuing to become the vas deferens. (From M. Dym (1977). In: *Histology*. 5th edn. Ed. by L. Weiss. Macmillan, London. Copyright by Elsevier Science Publishing Co., Inc.)

posteriorly through the abdomen, over the pelvic brim, to arrive in the scrotum. The innervation and blood supply of the testes consequently originate from the lumbar region and pass through the abdomen and the inguinal canal into the scrotum. The migration of the testes may go wrong; for example, one or both testes may fail to descend into the scrotum, resulting in *cryptorchidism* (literally 'hidden gonad'). Intra-abdominal testes are normal in some species (e.g. elephants and marine mammals), but are abnormal in the human. Species which normally have descended testes suffer from disorders of spermatogenesis if the testes fail to descend; the spermatogenic, but not the endocrine, function of the testes is arrested if testicular temperature is too high. The arrangement of the vascular supply to the testis, whereby the internal spermatic artery is coiled and passes through the spermatic cord very close to the pampiniform plexus draining venous blood from the testis, enables countercurrent heat exchange to occur between venous and arterial blood so keeping the testis cool. The underlying causes of (a) the temperature sensitivity of testicular function and/or (b) the extra-abdominal situation of the testes of many species, are obscure.

The testes of the fetus undergo a surge of endocrine activity which reaches a maximum during the 4th month of fetal life; the stimulus to this early activity, which is crucial for normal male sexual differentiation, is hCG secreted by the placenta. There is also a postnatal peak of testosterone secretion which is presumably the result of the temporary rise in pituitary gonadotrophin concentrations at this time, but the striking increase in testis size occurs at puberty when the endocrine activity of the interstitial cells of Leydig increases rapidly. The solid testicular cords develop a lumen and become tubules, the Sertoli cells increase in size and activity, and the germ cells resume mitotic activity.

The adult testes

Adult testes have endocrine and spermatogenic functions which are morphologically separate. The androgens are synthesized between the tubules, and the spermatozoa develop within the tubules. The extratubular fluids—the blood, and the interstitial fluid which is similar in composition to the lymph draining the testis—differ markedly in composition from the fluid in the lumen of the seminiferous tubule which contains more potassium, less sodium, less protein, hardly any immunoglobulins, less testosterone, no glucose, and more inositol.

A *blood-testis barrier* separates the compartments and consists of a multi-layered system of junctional complexes which completely surrounds each Sertoli cell and joins it to its neighbours (see Fig. 4.4). The fluid within the seminiferous tubule is produced largely by the Sertoli cells. Lying between the extratubular fluid compartment and the fluid within the lumen of the seminiferous tubule are two sub-compartments where most of the events of spermatogenesis take place: the *basal* compartment which is within the peritubular membrane but below the junctional complexes between the Sertoli cells, and the *adluminal* compartment which is within the tubule and is enclosed by the walls of neighbouring Sertoli cells; its base is formed by the junctional complexes between the Sertoli cells, and it communicates at its apex with the lumen of the tubule.

The endocrine function of the testis (Fig. 4.6)

The endocrine function of the testis is, first and foremost, to produce testosterone. This function is performed by the Leydig cells in the interstitial tissue of the testis; only these cells possess the 3,β-hydroxysteroid dehydrogenase which is needed for the $\Delta 5$ to $\Delta 4$ conversions needed for androgen synthesis (see Chapter 10). Most of the testosterone produced by the testis passes into testicular venous blood; a little passes into testicular lymph, and some passes into intratubular compartments of the testis. Testosterone, being fat-soluble, diffuses rapidly down a concentration gradient across the blood-testis barrier into the intratubular compartments of the testis; the free testosterone concentration within the tubules is reduced by binding to androgen receptors within target cells and to an androgen-binding protein (ABP) secreted by Sertoli cells which is found in the adluminal compartment and is similar to the testosterone-binding protein found in plasma. Testosterone not only has widespread effects on target organs outside the testis (see Chapter 10), but also has effects on spermatogenesis within the tubules.

The steroidogenic activity of the Leydig cells is controlled by luteinizing hormone (LH), which is subject to negative feedback control by plasma testosterone. LH secretion is also controlled by hypothalamic GnRH, and therefore by the brain and external environment. Although negative feedback control of LH by testosterone is the normal mode of steroid influence on LH secretion in the male, the pituitary gland of the male primate can be stimulated by exogenous oestradiol: if a sufficiently large dose is administered to men (particularly those with testicular failure) an initial inhibition of LH release is followed by a short-lived surge of plasma LH levels resembling the surge which causes ovulation in women.

Spermatogenesis

Spermatogenesis is the process which gives rise to mature spermatozoa. Spermatozoa are derived from testicular germ cells by a process involving *mitotic proliferation, meiosis* which produces genetic diversity and halves chromosome numbers, and *cell remodelling* (*spermiogenesis*) whereby the haploid cell is transformed into the mature state.

Mitosis in the germ cells of the testis is re-activated at the time of puberty, at which time the cells become known as *spermatogonia* (Fig. 4.3). Each spermatogonium undergoes a number of mitotic divisions which is characteristic for the species. In the rat, in which the process is best understood, there are six mitotic divisions. The original spermatogonium is known as 'A1' and successive products of mitosis are known as 'A2', 'A3', 'A4', 'intermediate spermatogonium', and finally 'spermatogonium Type B', each having a characteristic morphology. Some spermatogonia will not progress through all stages of this process, but give rise to new A1 spermatogonia to replace those which have differentiated; others degenerate at various stages of mitosis. The Type B spermatogonia undergo a final mitotic division to give rise to *primary spermatocytes* and these cells leave the basal compartment and somehow migrate through the tight junctions between neighbouring Sertoli cells into the adluminal compartment (Fig. 4.4). In this new environment they enter the first and prolonged meiotic prophase, during which shuffling of genetic information between paired homologous chromosomes occurs. This ensures genetic heterogeneity of spermatozoa, in spite of their derivation from genetically identical diploid cells. The first meiotic division yields two 'secondary spermatocytes', and these cells rapidly undergo a reduction division to yield two haploid 'early spermatids'. The various cell divisions described above are not complete, for strands of cytoplasm connect the almost-divided cells, and persist until the late spermatids are released into the lumen of the tubule as free spermatozoa.

Early spermatids have the chromosal content of the mature spermatozoon, but substantial remodelling (*spermiogenesis*) must occur before they reach maturity as spermatozoa (Fig. 4.5). The DNA of the spermatid becomes highly condensed, being packed into inactive units of chromatin together with

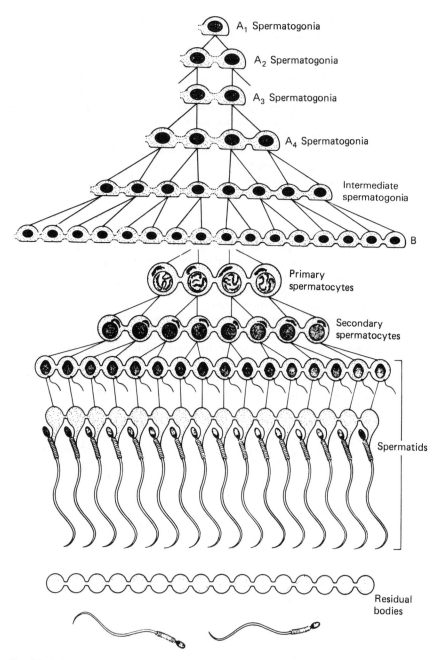

Fig. 4.3 A diagram illustrating the major cell types involved in spermatogenesis in the rat. Note the intercellular cytoplasmic bridges which connect almost-completely divided cells which are shown here in linear array, but which in reality form a tangled meshwork. (From Dym, M. and Fawcett, D.W. (1971). *Biology of Reproduction* **4**, 195–215.)

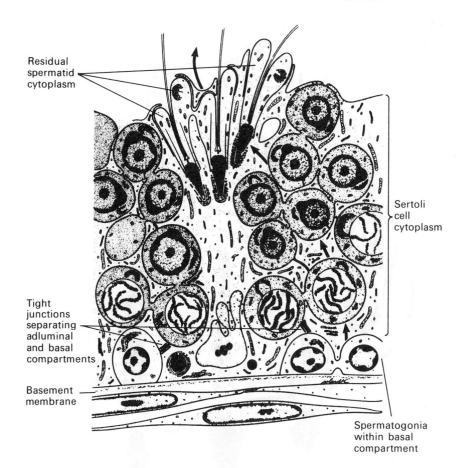

Residual spermatid cytoplasm

Sertoli cell cytoplasm

Tight junctions separating adluminal and basal compartments

Basement membrane

Spermatogonia within basal compartment

Fig. 4.4 Schematic representation of the seminiferous epithelium with a permanent population of columnar Sertoli cells, extending from the base to the free luminal surface, and a mobile population of germ cells, which occupy expanded intercellular spaces between neighbouring Sertoli cells and slowly move up their side as they pass through the successive stages of their differentiation into spermatozoa. (From Fawcett, D.W. (1974). In: *Male Fertility and Sterility*. Ed. by R.F. Mancini and L. Martini. Academic Press, New York.)

basic proteins which include lysine-rich histones; these sperm-specific histones seem to prevent gene expression, and are removed only after entry into the egg at fertilization. Spermiogenesis involves the generation of a *tail* (for propulsion), a *midpiece* containing mitochondria (for energy generation), the *acrosome* (which is packed with enzymes which will assist penetration into the egg), and the *residual body*. The whole process of spermatogenesis takes place in the immediate vicinity of, and is presumably influenced by, the Sertoli cells; the spermatids and their precursors in the adluminal and basal compartments indent the walls of the Sertoli cells and form specialized junctions with them.

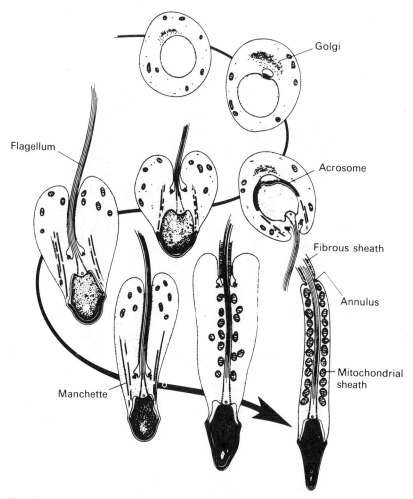

Fig. 4.5 A schematic drawing of the stages of spermiogenesis in the human starting with an early *spermatid* and ending with a *spermatozoon*. (From Dym, M. (1983). In: *Histology*. 5th edn. Ed. by L. Weiss. Macmillan, London. Copyright by Elsevier Science Publishing Co., Inc.)

As spermiogenesis proceeds, the differentiating cells move towards the lumen of the tubule. With the development of the sperm tail, junctional contacts with the spermatids and the Sertoli cells are lost, and the immature spermatids are released into the lumen of the tubule, where they are bathed in tubular fluid. They are carried away in this fluid through the various ducts of the testis to begin their journey towards the egg.

When any given A1 spermatogonium starts to divide, it generates daughter cells, one of which takes the place of the A1 spermatogonium which gave rise to it; this 'next generation' spermatogonium enters a period of quiescence, before starting to divide thereby initating a new cycle of spermatogenesis. The time interval between successive re-entries into spermatogenesis is one-quarter of the time taken for the completion of spermatogenesis, i.e. 16 days for the human. In any particular area of seminiferous tubular epithelium, four successive spermatogenic processes will therefore be occurring; the products of the earlier cycles of spermatogenesis will be displaced progressively towards the tubular lumen by the products of later cycles. A transverse section through the tubule will reveal spermatogenic cells at several stages of development, each type representing a point in a separate cycle. Since the cycle length, the total duration of spermatogenesis and the duration of each of its component stages are fixed, it follows that a spermatogenic cell at one particular stage of development will always be found in association (in a radial cross section) with other cells 16, 32, and 48 days further on in development. These fixed 'cell associations' are a striking feature of testicular histology. In most species, a particular cell association typically occupies an extensive area along the length of the seminiferous tubule, but in human tubules each association occupies a small patch of tubular epithelium, and does not extend around its circumference. A cross section through a human tubule can often reveal two to four different cell associations.

Hormonal control of spermatogenesis (Fig. 4.6)

The process of spermatogenesis takes a certain time which is fixed and characteristic for any particular species (64 days in man). Hormones can alter the number of spermatogonia advancing through spermatogenesis, but they do not affect the rate at which the process occurs. Spermatogenesis does not proceed beyond the primary spermatocyte stage after hypophysectomy, and type A spermatogonia decrease in number. Replacement of LH restores spermatogenesis to some extent, but not the number of germ cells. The prime site of action of LH is the interstitial (Leydig) cell of the testis where it regulates testosterone secretion, and the effects of LH on spermatogenesis are mediated by testosterone. The prime site of action of FSH is the Sertoli cell, where synthesis of protein—in particular, specific proteins such as androgen-binding protein—is increased; however, FSH may also stimulate the mitotic activity of spermatogonia. Secretion of FSH and LH from the anterior pituitary gland is influenced by a range of factors including external environmental influences (see Chapter 2) as well as negative feedback effects exerted by testosterone and 'inhibin' (see Chapter 10).

Sperm maturation

Tubular fluid in the testis is the product of the Sertoli cells, and flows from the tubules towards the rete testis laden with immature spermatozoa. The fluid alters in composition as it passes through the rete testis, and further changes occur in the vasa efferentia and the epididymis, where carnitine, glycerylphosphorylcholine and various glycoproteins are added. Much of the fluid is absorbed in the epididymis leading to a 100-fold increase in sperm concentration. As their fluid environment changes from the rete testis, via vasa efferentia and epididymis to the vas deferens—a journey which takes about 12 days—so the spermatozoa develop the capacity to swim and to

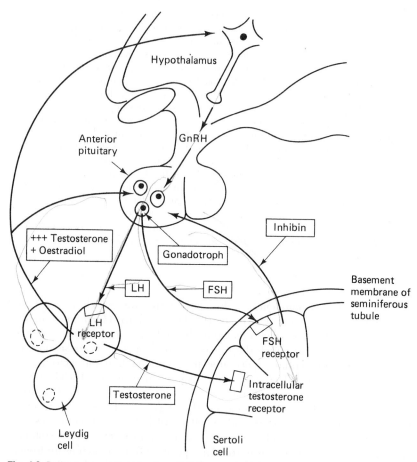

Fig. 4.6 Pathways by which the hypothalamus and pituitary control of the two major testicular functions, steroid secretion (left) and spermatogenesis (right). Luteinizing hormone binds exclusively to testicular Leydig cells causing them to secrete testosterone and, to a lesser extent, oestradiol. These steroids exert negative feedback control of gonadotrophin release. Testosterone secreted by Leydig cells binds to cytoplasmic receptors in Sertoli cells and acts upon them, as does FSH, to influence spermatogenesis. Inhibin from Sertoli cells reduces FSH secretion.

fertilize. The process of nuclear condensation is completed, the residual body migrates down the tail and is discarded, and there are also small changes in the structure of the acrosome. The structure of the mature spermatozoon is shown in Fig. 4.7. These maturational processes require adequate stimulation of the epididymis by androgens, which are delivered by fluid in the rete testis containing a high concentration of testosterone bound to androgen-binding protein, together with a lower concentration of dihydrotestosterone. The testosterone enters the cells of the epididymis, undergoes conversion by 5α-reductase to DHT, and is bound to cytoplasmic receptors; activated DHT-

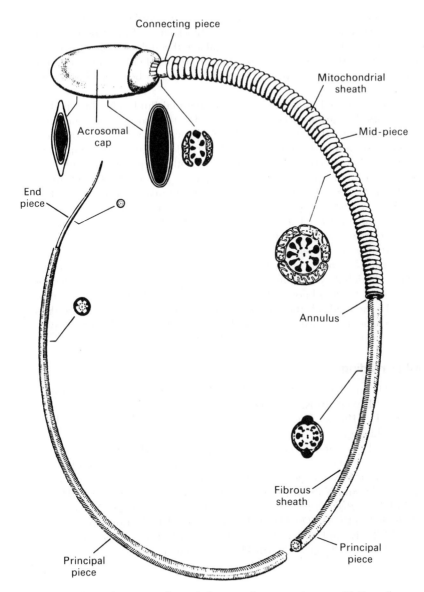

Fig. 4.7 The internal structure of a typical mammalian spermatozoon with the cell membrane removed. Its total length is about 60 × 10⁻⁶ metres. (From Fawcett, D.W. (1975). *Development Biology* **44**, 394.)

receptor complexes are then translocated to the nuclei where they bring about the metabolic processes necessary for sperm maturation.

As spermatozoa pass from the tail of the epididymis into the vas deferens they are densely packed and are propelled slowly by the muscular activity of the epididymis and vas deferens. No large fluid flow occurs in this region, and after ligation of the vas (*vasectomy*) no large accumulation of fluid occurs, though spermatozoa build up behind the blockage and must be removed by phagocytosis within the epididymis or leakage through its wall. Normally the vas serves to store spermatozoa and they are released either at ejaculation or, if this does not occur, by oozing into the urethra to be washed away in the urine.

Semen is composed of spermatozoa and seminal fluid. The fluid is derived largely from the various accessory sex glands—the prostate, seminal vesicles, and bulbo-urethral (Cowper's) gland—and provides a vehicle for transporting the spermatozoa into the female tract. A normal human semen sample has the following characteristics: volume—1.5–5 ml (typically about 3 ml); spermatozoa—at least 20 000 000/ml (typically about 100 000 000/ml); not more than 25 per cent of spermatozoa with abnormal structure, and more than 30 per cent showing progressive motility. Human seminal fluid includes, fructose (at least 1.5 mg/ml), inositol (0.4 mg/ml), citric acid (0.1–0.3 mg/ml), acid phosphatase, glycerylphosphorylcholine (0.5 mg/ml), and prostaglandins. Spermatozoa taken directly from the vas deferens can fertilize eggs, so none of these added ingredients are essential for sperm function, though they presumably contribute to the nutrition and protection of spermatozoa. Little is known about the normal physiology of the accessory sex glands. To the medical student, their importance derives largely from the fact that one of them, the prostate, can enlarge either by benign hypertrophy or as a result of cancer, and cause urinary obstruction.

Further reading

Burger, H. and Kretser, D. de (eds) (1981). *Comprehensive Endocrinology: The Testis*. Raven Press, New York.

Daggett, P. (1981). The testis. Chap. 8 in *Clinical Endocrinology*. Edward Arnold, London.

Hamilton, D.W. and Greep, R.O. (eds) (1975). *Male Reproductive System*. Volume V of Section 7 (Endocrinology) of the Handbook of Physiology. American Physiological Society, Washington, D.C.

Hamilton, D. and Naftolin, F. (eds) (1982). *Reproductive Function in Men*. Vol. 2 of *Basic Reproductive Medicine*, MIT Press, Cambridge, Mass.

Setchell, B.P. (1978). *The Mammalian Testis*. Paul Elek, London.

Spring-Mills, E. and Hafez, E.S.E. (1980). *Male Accessory Sex Glands: Biology and Pathology*. Elsevier-North Holland, New York.

5

Coming together

Reproductive behaviour

The physiological mechanisms which ensure the production of male and female gametes in a state of readiness for fertilization would be useless if coitus and the behaviour leading up to it did not occur. 'Reproductive fitness' (a concept introduced to describe the overall capacity of an individual to reproduce offspring which will themselves attain sexual maturity) is a function both of proper functioning of the gonads, uterus, seminal vesicles and so on, and also of behaviour such as courtship, copulation and rearing.

We have discussed in Chapter 1 the differentiation of the reproductive system in the male, including a brief reference to the development of male behaviour. Penile erections are seen during rapid-eye-movement sleep in male infants, and masturbation leading to orgasm, but without ejaculation, is the rule rather than the exception in adolescent boys; nocturnal erections and ejaculations are normal throughout adult life in the male. Comparable phenomena in females are less well documented.

Control of sexual behaviour

Libido (from the Latin word meaning 'lust') is increased by androgens in men and women. It is manifested both as fantasy and as behavioural activity. There is, however, no simple link between sexual activity and circulating hormone levels. We have seen how environmental stimuli, including sexual activity itself, may influence sex hormone secretion—and the reciprocity between sexual behaviour and sex hormones secretion must be emphasized.

The dependence of male sexual and/or aggressive behaviour on androgens is demonstrable by its marked decline after castration, and restoration by administration of testosterone. Testosterone disappears from the plasma within hours of castration, but the decline in sexual behaviour may take days or weeks. Restoration of male behaviour after testosterone treatment is similarly sluggish. The behavioural effect of androgens may be due at least in part to their effects on the tactile sensitivity of peripheral target tissues, e.g. the penis, as opposed to direct effects on the brain itself. Anti-androgens, such as cyproterone acetate, decrease sexual arousal. Oestrogens given to men cause regression of the penis, testes and prostate gland, together with impotence and loss of ability to ejaculate.

Sexual behaviour in female non-primates is strictly dependent on steroid hormones and a limited period of sexual receptivity ('oestrus' or 'heat') is closely co-ordinated with ovulation so as to ensure that fertilization occurs. Animals like the cat, which are reflex ovulators, come into heat and stay in that state until coitus—and therefore ovulation—occurs. These behavioural changes are a direct consequence of the action of ovarian steroids on the brain. Ovarian hormones have little direct effect on libido in women, but androgens of adrenal origin may increase it (see p. 47).

Environmental stimuli also exert a direct effect on sexual behaviour. Olfactory attractants are important in species as widely different as insects and monkeys; there is little scientific evidence of their importance in the human, but subjective experience, and perfume sales, support the notion that smell can contribute to the attractiveness of a sexual partner. Physical appearance clearly influences sexual attractiveness in men and women, though its influence is profoundly affected by fashion and by individual perceptual differences. The tactile stimulation of body contact, particularly of certain parts of the body (the *erogenous zones*) including the clitoris, inner thighs, nipples and ear lobes, can under appropriate circumstances act in concert with other stimuli to create a high level of sexual excitement.

Coitus, and the human sexual response

Sexual excitement leads to an observable physical sexual response in both men and women which has been described and codified by Masters and Johnson. They described a series of essentially arbitrary stages in the process of sexual arousal which are summarized in Table 5.1. The events described are complex responses mediated by both autonomic and somatic motor systems; they are influenced by many sensory modalities, and are particularly dependent on input from mechanoreceptors in the perineal region. Coitus may be undertaken in a variety of positions, with the face-to-face position with the man above (the 'missionary position') being the most common. Coitus tends to decrease in frequency as pregnancy advances, though there are few contra-indications to coitus during pregnancy, except perhaps in early pregnancy in women who habitually abort.

The pursuit of the intense pleasure normally encountered in satisfactory sexual intercourse motivates much human behaviour, though the neural mechanisms are obscure. The physiology of pleasure is no clearer than the physiology of pain. Consideration and affection for the partner, experience, age, health, privacy, fatigue, technique, and lack of worry are amongst the factors which affect the physiology, the subjective sensation and the frequency of coitus. A full and considerate sexual life can enhance the quality of human relationships; conversely sexual inadequacy can be a major contributor to their breakdown (Steele: *Gynaecology, Obstetrics and the Neonate*, Chapter 20).

Homosexuality

Homosexuality is a term which can be used to describe either a sexual behavioural act between individuals of the same gender, or a more or less

Table 5.1 The characteristics of the four stages of the sexual response cycle described by Masters and Johnson

Stage 1: Excitement: Increase in respiration, pulse rate, blood pressure; may last from minutes to an hour or more.

Male
Erection of penis caused by vasocongestion of corpora cavernosa.
Blood flow into the penis rises but flow *through* the penis does not because the vein draining the penis is compressed.
Thickening of scrotal skin due to activity of the dartos muscle.

Female
Erection of nipple and enlargement of areola.
Doubling of size of clitoris.
Swelling of labia minora.
Reddening and enlargement of labia minora.
Appearance of vaginal transudate.
Expansion of vaginal cavity.
Elevation of uterus.

Stage 2: Plateau: Lasts from one to several minutes. Further increase in respiration, heart rate, and blood presure (increase of 20–40 mmHg).

Male
Full penile erection.
Full elevation and increase in size of the testes due to vaso-congestion.
Appearance of an emission from tip of penis containing some viable spermatozoa; this emission which occurs prior to orgasm, can account for the failure of 'coitus interruptus' as a contraceptive method.

Female
Skin becomes flushed.
Breast size increases.
Retraction of shaft of clitoris.
Swelling and opening of labia minora.
Copious vaginal transudate.
Continued ballooning of upper two-thirds of vagina, but swelling of outer third to form 'orgasmic platform' (the contracted region providing increased traction on the thrusting penis). Further elevation and contraction of the uterus.
Hyperventilation and carpopedal spasm.

Stage 3: Orgasm: Lasts only 3–15 seconds. Its physiology and associated subjective sensations are highly variable. Some of the following features may occur: 3–12 generalised contractions of pelvic musculature including sphincters, penis, vagina, uterus, and also much of the body musculature producing facial grimaces. Blood pressure may rise by 40–100 mmHg systolic, and 20–50 mmHg diastolic. Heart rate can increase to 180/min, and respiration to 40/min. In both male and female, the endpoint is equally definite; in the male it is marked by ejaculation of 3–5 ml of semen. Orgasm culminates in a sense of quiet euphoria and total relaxation.

Male
Subjective sensation that ejaculation cannot be averted.
Then sensation of semen entering urethra as accessory organs contract to force it forward. Next experience of violent contractions of pelvic musculature which, later, can be voluntarily controlled.

Female
Orgasm initiated by an instant 'suspended sensation' followed by a surge of sexual awareness. Consciousness is enveloped in the experience, and this is followed by a suffusion of warmth from the pelvis throughout the body. The experience of orgasm in the female is continuously subject to interference by psychological disturbance (e.g. a fleeting doubt or an unexpected noise in the next room).

Stage 4: Resolution: 'Detumescence' as blood is disgorged from the genitalia. Physiological indices return to the resting state. Resolution takes a matter of minutes after orgasm, but may take several hours if orgasm has not been attained.

Male
There is an absolute refractory period following orgasm during which a second orgasm cannot be attained. It tends to increase with age from minutes to as much as 24 hours.

Female
The mature female is capable of multiple orgasms in rapid succession.

enduring erotic predisposition by an individual for others of the same gender. Homosexual behaviour is found in many animals, and has existed amongst male and female humans throughout recorded history and in all parts of the world. It may take many forms. Its genesis is not understood. It is probably both unjustifiable and unhelpful to regard it as either a disease or as abnormal. Some male homosexuals are promiscuous, and consequently run a high risk of sexually transmissible diseases.

Transport and development of spermatozoa in the female tract

The occurrence of coitus leaves semen deposited within the vagina. The semen coagulates into a gelatinous material as a result of the action of coagulating enzymes derived from the prostate on a fibrinogen-like substrate from the seminal vesicle. The coagulate is then gradually dissolved by the activation of a proenzyme derived from the prostate.

Once within the female, the first hurdle facing the spermatozoa is passage from the vagina through the cervix into the uterus. It is possible for sperm to achieve this only during a limited period of 'oestrogen-dominance' in mid-menstrual-cycle when the physical characteristics of the cervical mucus are favourable. During the follicular phase of the cycle, the mucus increases in quantity, and immediately before ovulation it is profuse and clear. It then becomes thick and viscous, and therefore difficult to penetrate, during the luteal phase. Regular low dosage with progestagens ('mini-pills') may achieve its contraceptive effect by creating an impenetrable cervical mucus throughout the cycle without preventing ovulation (Steele: *Gynaecology, Obstetrics and the Neonate*, Chapter 15). Physical tests can be applied to cervical mucus: when its condition is most favourable to sperm penetration it can be stretched relatively far before the threads snap (a high 'Spinnbarkeit'), and if allowed to dry on a microscope slide, it forms a characteristic ferning pattern.

Most spermatozoa fail to enter the uterus and leak from the vagina. The minority that enter the uterus traverse it quite rapidly and are found in the human oviduct just a few minutes after copulation. After coitus, spermatozoa can survive for several days; they retain their fertility in the oviduct for up to 48 hours, and may survive even longer in the uterine glands or the cervix. Transport of spermatozoa through the uterus results from peristaltic contractions of its wall, which may be enhanced (i) by oxytocin released from the neurohypophysis of the woman at the time of coitus, and (ii) by prostaglandins present in the seminal plasma. Of the millions of spermatozoa in a normal ejaculate, only a small proportion reach the ampulla of the oviduct which is the site of fertilization. Some get even further, passing via the fimbrial end of the oviduct into the peritoneal cavity.

Capacitation

If spermatozoa recovered from an ejaculate are examined, they swim vigorously and appear to be mature. However, if placed with eggs in vitro, they either do not fertilize them, or do so only after a delay. Spermatozoa recovered from the uterus or oviduct a few hours after coitus are, by contrast, capable of immediate fertilization. Something must therefore happen to the spermatozoa within the female tract which leads to their attaining the *capacity* to fertilize, and that something has been termed *capacitation*. No readily identifiable morphological changes can be detected during the process, but some subtle alteration occurs in the spermatozoal membrane—probably involving the removal of surface coats—which alters the behaviour of the membrane and enables the spermatozoa to undergo the next stage in the process of fertilization. No single agent within the uterus or oviduct accounts for capacitation, and it can be induced in vitro by culture solutions of simple composition.

Activation: the acrosome reaction

After capacitation, the spermatozoa must become *activated* before they can fertilize. The most striking component of the process of activation is the *acrosome reaction*. The acrosome is a vesicle which forms a cap around the apex of the sperm head. The inner membrane of the acrosome lies adjacent to the nuclear membrane of the spermatozoon, and the outer membrane lies immediately under the plasma membrane. The acrosome reaction probably results from an instability in the surface membrane of the front of the spermatozoon somehow induced by the proximity of the oocyte. Movement of calcium ions across the plasma membrane seems to be involved in the acrosome reaction, the morphological changes in which have much in common with the process of 'stimulus-secretion coupling' involved in, for example, the release of neurotransmitters at nerve terminals, where calcium is also important. The plasma membrane at the front of the spermatozoon fuses at several sites with the underlying acrosomal membrane (Fig. 5.1) thereby exposing the contents of the acrosomal vesicle to the exterior. At the same time, the movements of the tail of the spermatozoon change from an undulating wave-like pattern to a more episodic large-amplitude 'whiplash' pattern. At about the same time there is also a change in the plasma membrane in the more posterior part of the sperm head, whereby it becomes capable of fusing with the surface membrane of the egg.

Fertilization

In Chapter 3 (p. 38) we left the egg immediately after ovulation. The oocyte, with attached cumulus cells, is picked up by the fimbria at the ostium of the oviduct and swept by cilia along the ampulla towards the isthmus. In the ampulla, the oocyte and the spermatozoa meet and after the activation of the spermatozoa, fertilization begins. The oocyte will die if it is not fertilized fairly soon after ovulation; estimates of its lifespan in the human range from 6 to 24 hours.

The contents released from the spermatozoon as a result of the acrosome reaction include the enzyme *hyaluronidase*. This digests the intercellular cement which holds the cumulus cells together, enabling the spermatozoon to reach the zona pellucida. Here the spermatozoon attaches to receptors, and lies flat on the surface of the membrane. These receptors on the zona pellucida are almost species-specific, and as fertilization proceeds their properties change—the *zona reaction*—as a result of which they will bind no further spermatozoa. The spermatozoon passes obliquely through the zona, aided by its whiplash tail movements, along a pathway which is thought to be digested by a lysin (*acrosin*) bound to the acrosomal membrane. Thus it comes to lie in the *perivitelline space* between the zona and the *vitelline membrane* of the oocyte. The membrane of the sperm head then fuses with the vitelline membrane (Fig. 5.1) and movements of the spermatozoon cease. When the sperm head attaches to the vitelline membrane, calcium ions enter the cytoplasm of the oocyte, and the cortical vesicles which lie just beneath the vitelline membrane disappear (Fig. 5.1) and their contents pass into the perivitelline space

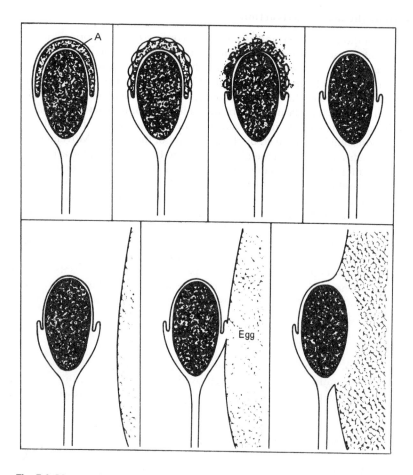

Fig. 5.1 Diagram showing the pattern of the acrosome reaction and the early steps in sperm-egg fusion during which exocytosis of cortical vesicles, which lie just below the vitelline membrane, results in release of their contents into the perivitelline space. The granulosa cells surrounding the egg, and the zona pellucida, have been omitted from this diagram. (A = acrosome) (Drawn by J.R. Fuller from Austin, C.R. (1972). In: *Germ Cells and Fertilization*. Book 1 of Reproduction in Mammals. Ed. by C.R. Austin and R.V. Short. Cambridge University Press, Cambridge.)

('stimulus-secretion coupling' again). Among these contents are enzymes which act on the zona to cause the zona reaction whereby further penetration of spermatozoa is impaired. This constitutes one mechanism which ensures that each oocyte is fertilized by only one spermatozoon, i.e. the *block to polyspermy*.

The fusion of sperm and egg membranes is followed by the sinking of the sperm head into the cytoplasm of the ovum, the reactivation of meiotic metaphase and the extrusion of the second polar body. The sperm head forms a male pronucleus. Nucleoli appear and a new nuclear envelope is formed. Deoxyribonucleic acid (DNA) is now replicated and transcription of maternal and paternal genes begins. The pronuclear membranes around the reduplicated sets of parental chromosomes break down, the metaphase spindle forms, and the chromosomes assume their positions at its equator. *Syngamy*, i.e. the coming together of the chromosomes of the paternal and maternal gametes, has now been achieved and the ovum has become a *zygote*. Anaphase and telophase follow, the cleavage furrow forms and the two-cell *embryo* results.

Early development of the embryo (Fig. 5.2)

The embryo remains within the oviduct for about three and a half days after coitus, and is then transferred through the isthmus to the uterus. Rising progesterone levels in the luteal phase of the cycle are responsible for relaxing the musculature of the oviduct, uterotubal junction, and uterus, thereby facilitating this journey. The cilia of the oviduct play an important part in embryo transport, and are responsible for moving the embryo in the right direction. Within the oviduct, early embryonic development occurs. Each of the two cells in the early embryo undergoes a series of divisions known as *cleavage* during which its total size does not change; this process yields a *morula*—the name given to the embryo between about the 8 to the 32 cell stage. Synthesis of RNA and protein is increasing rapidly at this stage which is reached about three and a half days after ovulation. The appearance of the fluid-filled *blastocoelic cavity* marks the transition from morula to *blastocyst*; at this stage, which is reached shortly after the morula arrives in the uterine lumen, differentiation of cell types is first seen in the embryo: (a) an outer layer of *trophectoderm* or *trophoblast*, cells of which are not destined to form part of the developing fetus, but do contribute to the formation of the placenta and fetal membranes, and (b) eccentrically placed at one pole of the cavity, a cluster of cells, the *inner cell mass*, which will give rise to the fetus. The term *conceptus* includes *both* the fetus *and* the other structures originally derived from the fertilized egg.

At the late-morula stage, transfer from the oviduct into the uterus occurs. If this transfer occurs too early, the morula will enter a hostile uterine environment and further development will fail. If embryo transfer from the oviduct into the uterus should fail, implantation into the wall of the oviduct may result giving rise to *tubal pregnancy*. The early blastocyst, normally within the uterus, develops initially within the zona pellucida and this is shed about 6 days after fertilization by a process which may involve a combination of 'hatching' (as a grape skin is peeled from a grape) and digestion by uterine

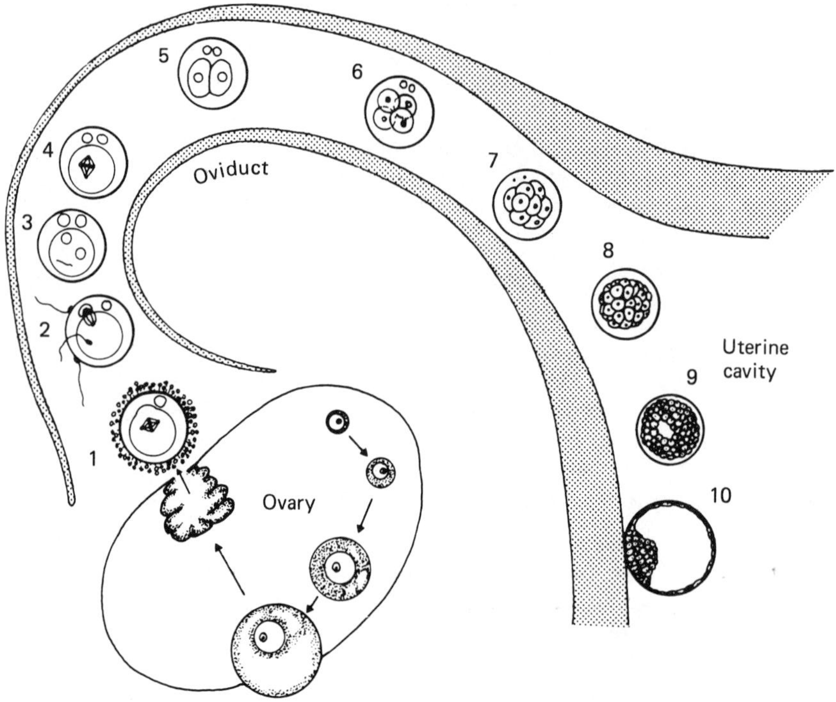

Key

1: Egg released from ovary with first polar body and second metaphase spindle

2: Sperm entry into egg, second polar body forming

3: Male and female pronucleus formation. Sperm tail in egg cytoplasm

4: First cleavage metaphase spindle

5: 2-cell stage

6: 4-cell stage

7: 8-cell stage

8: Morula

9: Early blastocyst, blastocoele cavity forming

10: Blastocyst starting to implant

Fig. 5.2 Diagrammatic representation of follicular growth, ovulation, fertilization and embryonic development prior to implantation. (From Whittingham, D.G. (1979). *British Medical Bulletin* **35**, 105–111.)

Fig. 5.3 The process of implantation. In (a) a blastocyst is seen in the early stage of implantation. In (b) development has proceeded and uterine epithelium has almost completely regrown over the implanting embryo, i.e. 'interstitial' implantation. (From Tuchmann-Duplessis, H., David, G. and Haegel, P. (1971). *Illustrated Human Embryology*, vol. 1. Springer-Verlag, New York; Chapman and Hall, London; Masson et Cie, Paris.)

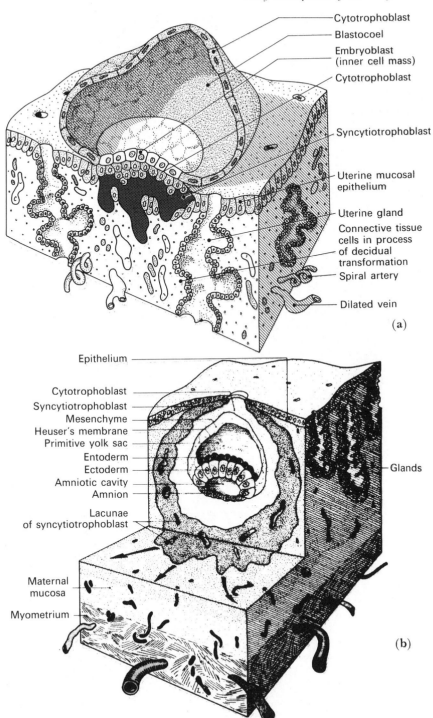

Cytotrophoblast
Blastocoel
Embryoblast
(inner cell mass)
Cytotrophoblast

Syncytiotrophoblast

Uterine mucosal
epithelium

Uterine gland
Connective tissue
cells in process
of decidual
transformation
Spiral artery

Dilated vein

(a)

Epithelium

Cytotrophoblast
Syncytiotrophoblast
Mesenchyme
Heuser's membrane
Primitive yolk sac
Entoderm
Ectoderm
Amniotic cavity
Amnion

Lacunae
of syncytiotrophoblast

Glands

Maternal
mucosa

Myometrium

(b)

lytic agents e.g. protease (Fig. 5.4). Prior to implantation, the blastocyst obtains its metabolic requirements from *uterine milk*: a mixture of endometrial secretions and tissue debris. Meanwhile the endometrium, under the influence of rising maternal progesterone levels, is undergoing the changes characteristic of the secretory phase of the endometrial cycle (see p. 45).

Implantation (Fig. 5.3)

Implantation begins when the blastocyst makes contact with the endometrium; this most often occurs on the posterior wall of the body of the uterus. Only a few trophoblast cells make the initial contact with the uterine epithelium, yet within an hour stromal tissue underlying the epithelium shows evidence of modifications of structure and function. These are presumably due to some signal from the conceptus. Various substances have been suggested as the specific inducer of these changes—including histamine, carbon dioxide, prostaglandins and oestradiol. However, a maternal endometrial response similar to that provoked by a blastocyst can be triggered in many species by non-specific stimuli such as glass beads or mild trauma. The modification in the uterine stromal tissue during implantation is known as *decidualization*; initially there is an increase in the vascular permeability of the tissue, followed by oedema, changes in the composition of the intercellular matrix, alterations in the structure of the stromal cells, and a progressive increase in capillary density. The process prepares the tissue which will form the major endometrial component of the placenta which, since it will eventually be shed like leaves from a tree, is known as the *decidua*.

A few hours after implantation begins, the uterine epithelium underlying the point of contact with the blastocyst becomes eroded, apparently by invading trophoblast cells. As the trophoblast invades, some of its cells fuse together forming *syncytiotrophoblast*, while others retain their individual cell walls to form a tissue known as *cytotrophoblast*. The invasion of the uterine glandular tissue and of the underlying stroma results in the release of large amounts of metabolic substrate (lipids, carbohydrates, nucleic acid and proteins) which undergo digestion by the trophoblast cells; the products pass in the rapidly developing blood vascular system to the developing embryo.

The extent to which the conceptus invades the endometrium varies from species to species; in man the conceptus invades the maternal tissue so deeply that the uterine surface epithelium becomes restored over it—*interstitial* implantation. As the invasion of maternal tissue proceeds, the maternal blood vessels are eroded so that the trophoblast cells are bathed in maternal blood, forming a *haemo-chorial* placenta. In other species, the number of layers of tissue between the circulation of the mother and that of the conceptus is greater, but there seems to be no systematic link between the number of such layers and the efficiency of placental exchange.

Hormones play a part in controlling implantation; evidence for this comes from studies of *delayed implantation* in species such as the badger and the red deer, in which the blastocyst may lie dormant in the uterus for some months. Oestrogens may stimulate implantation in these species, and also in man. Some of these oestrogens could be of ovarian origin, because the time when

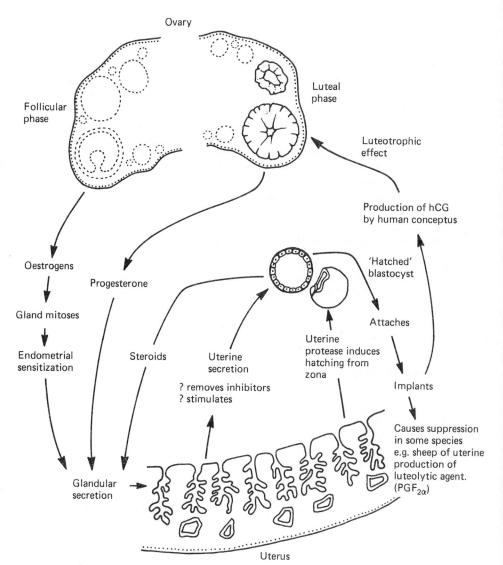

Fig. 5.4 A summary of the interactions between maternal and embryonic tissue which occur early in a pregnancy. The sequence begins with ovulation and sensitization of the uterus, and ends with hatching, attachment and implantation of the blastocyst, and maintenance of the corpus luteum by hormones of embryonic origin—notably hCG. (Modified from drawing by J.R. Fuller in Renfree, M.B. (1982). In: *Embryonic and Fetal Development*. Book 2 of Reproduction in Mammals, 2nd edn. Ed. by C.R. Austin and R.V. Short. Cambridge University Press, Cambridge.)

implantation occurs (about 6 days after ovulation) coincides with a modest postovulatory rise in oestrogen secretion from the corpus luteum (see Fig. 3.7). It is also possible that the conceptus itself synthesizes oestrogens which stimulate the progesterone-primed uterus. There must be synchrony between the age of the embryo and the stage of endometrial development if implantation is to be successful, and this may be partly related to the need for an optimal endocrine environment for the endometrium.

The intra-uterine device (IUD) probably exerts its 'contraceptive' effect at or about the time of implantation. The mechanism of its action is not yet established, but possibilities include: (i) interference with tubal transport of ova and embryos, (ii) prevention of implantation by creating a hostile uterine environment by, for example, provoking an inflammatory reaction in the endometrium, and (iii) early abortion *after* an early form of implantation (Steele: *Gynaecology, Obstetrics and the Neonate*, Chapter 15).

Maternal recognition of the onset of pregnancy

With the embryo safely implanted in the wall of the uterus, pregnancy can be regarded as well under way. The maintenance of pregnancy requires the prolongation of the lifespan of the corpus luteum. The mechanism by which this is achieved is discussed in the next chapter, but a summary of the mechanisms underlying interactions between conceptus, uterus and corpus luteum is given in Fig. 5.4.

Further reading

Ciba Foundation Symposium No. 64 (1978). *Maternal Recognition of Pregnancy*. Excerpta Medica, Amsterdam.

Edwards, R.G. and Purdy, J.M. (eds) (1981). *Human Conception In Vitro*. Academic Press, London.

Gagnon, J.H. (1977). *Human Sexualities*. Scott, Foresman and Company, Glenview, Illinois.

Gwatkin, R.B.L. (1977). *Fertilization Mechanisms in Man and Mammals*. Plenum Press, New York.

Masters, W.H. and Johnson, V.E. (1966). *Human Sexual Response*. Little Brown and Company, Boston.

Tuchmann-Duplessis, H., David, G. and Haegal, P. (1980). *Embryogenesis*. Vol. 1 of *Illustrated Human Embryology*. Chapman and Hall, London.

6

Pregnancy

The placenta

Mammalian reproduction is unique in offering a prolonged period of protection to the young, and this is maximized in the earliest stages of development by retaining the fetus within the uterus. The function of the *placenta* is to make this intrauterine pregnancy possible. It does this in many ways, e.g. by serving as a site for transport and diffusion between fetal and maternal blood, by secreting hormones, by protecting the fetus from maternal immunological attack, and by synthesizing and storing nutrients.

The development of the placenta

Initially the nutritional and waste-disposal needs of the conceptus are met by transport from, or diffusional exchange with, the fluids secreted by uterine glands. The growth and secretory activity of the glandular endometrium of the uterus is enhanced by the relatively high levels of progesterone produced by the ovary during the days following ovulation. This method of nutrition and waste-disposal can serve the needs of the conceptus for only a short time, and the conceptus soon develops its own blood vascular system to assist the distribution of vital metabolites being absorbed at its surface. A particular part of the surface becomes well vascularized, and this area enlarges by the devlopment of branching villi. These villi, composed of fetal tissue, become filled with thin walled capillaries and invade the maternal tissue during implantation (see p. 69).

Implantation culminates in the breakdown of maternal tissue so that the fetal villi eventually come to dip into large lakes (or *sinusoids*) of maternal blood. A placenta of *discoid* shape is formed and the endothelial wall of the fetal capillary is separated from the maternal blood by just a single layer of fetal *chorionic trophoblast* tissue. This tissue is characterized by cells fused together to form *syncytiotrophoblast*. A placental interface between maternal blood and a single layer of fetal chorionic tissue is classified as *haemochorial*. By comparison with many other species, the human placenta shows a high degree of invasion of maternal tissue by the fetus, and there are therefore fewer tissue layers separating fetal and maternal circulations.

On the fetal side of the established placenta (Fig. 6.1) there are about 60 branched villi. The floor of the placenta has many projections (*septa*) which are

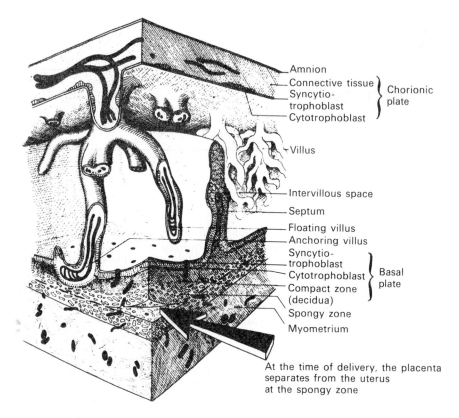

Amnion
Connective tissue
Syncytio-
trophoblast
Cytotrophoblast
} Chorionic plate

Villus

Intervillous space
Septum
Floating villus
Anchoring villus
Syncytio-
trophoblast
Cytotrophoblast
Compact zone
(decidua)
} Basal plate
Spongy zone
Myometrium

At the time of delivery, the placenta
separates from the uterus
at the spongy zone

Fig. 6.1 The structure of the mature placenta. At the time of delivery the placenta separates from the uterus at the spongy zone marked by the arrow. (From Tuchmann-Duplessis, H., David, G. and Haegel, P. (1971). *Illustrated Human Embryology*, vol. 1. Springer-Verlag, New York; Chapman and Hall, London; Masson et Cie, Paris.)

formed from maternal decidual tissue; these divide the maternal surface into about 20 lobes each of which contain several fetal villi.

Placental blood supply

There are two placental circulations, connected in parallel to the systemic circulations of mother and fetus. Maternal placental blood flow rate is less than the flow rate in the maternal uterine artery, because much of the blood in that artery supplies the rest of the uterus. Flow in the fetal placental circulation, however, is equal to that in the umbilical arteries or veins. Maternal blood reaching the placenta passes initially through about 100 spiral or convoluted arteries which open at the base of the septa, or at the apices of low conical projections of decidua; this causes a fall in hydrostatic pressure leading to a reduction in velocity of flow as the blood passes from these arteries into wide placental sinuses which form the *intervillous spaces* between the fetal villi. In order to leave these spaces, the blood must perfuse through a densely packed mass of villi through interstices which resemble a capillary bed. Thence blood passes to the 'extralobular' space, which is relatively free of villi, and drains through venous openings in the decidual plate of the placenta. Although there are no maternal blood vessels in the intervillous space, one can conceive of arterial, capillary and venous areas. Indeed there is a pressure gradient between the centres of the lobes and the extralobular spaces.

Maternal blood flow to the uterus as a whole rises linearly throughout pregnancy to about 500–750 ml/min at term. About 75 per cent of this reaches the intervillous space. Expressed in terms of rate of blood flow per kilogram of fetal weight, uterine blood flow decreases substantially towards the end of pregnancy. Resistance vessels in the uterus are dilated by exogenous administration of oestrogens, histamine and acetylcholine, and are constricted by progesterone, adrenaline and noradrenaline. Angiotensin II, which is produced by placental renin, may also influence uterine blood flow. Uterine blood flow is doubled in twin pregnancies.

On the fetal side, tortuous arterial branches supply the capillaries of the villi; the capillaries have a much larger cross-sectional area than the arteries and possess sinusoid-like expansions. Thus there are specializations on both fetal and maternal sides of the interface which facilitate placental exchange.

Transport of substances between maternal and fetal circulation

The placenta as a barrier
The maternal and fetal circulations are almost, but not quite, independent. Fetal erythrocytes are detectable in the maternal circulation in about half the mothers investigated, with the incidence of detection increasing as pregnancy advances. Maternal erythrocytes much less commonly enter the fetal circulation. Fetal trophoblast cells are frequently found in the maternal circulation and may colonize maternal tissues; their presence is normally benign, but can be malignant (choriocarcinoma). Cellular leakage may occur through minute ruptures in villous vessels, and is more likely to occur if pressure within fetal capillaries rises due to an increase of fetal venous resistance. Although the imperfections in the barrier are slight, with cell transfer amounting to only a fraction of a millilitre per day, this small transfer is enough to be of immunological significance; antigens on fetal cells may provoke the production of maternal antibodies — the basis of *haemolytic disease of the newborn.*

Much of our knowledge of the permeability of the placenta to water and solutes has been derived from the use of the *diffusion equilibrium technique.* A test substance is infused into a chronically catheterized sheep fetus until an equilibrium condition is reached when the rate of transplacental diffusion is equal to the rate of infusion. Using this method it is found that the transplacental movement of water and antipyrine is limited only by the rate of fetal placental blood flow, and is thus described as 'flow-limited'. Urea movement is partly limited by the permeability of the placental membrane, and movement of both sodium and chloride is greatly limited by low permeability of the placental membrane; the movement of such substances is described as 'membrane-limited'. In general the placenta presents less of a barrier to the free movement of lipid-soluble molecules than to large water-soluble molecules; the latter, if they do cross the placenta, do so with the assistance of specific mechanisms, i.e. by active transport or facilitated diffusion.

Blood gases

The placenta serves as the fetal lung. Its efficiency in that role, expressed as diffusion rate of gases per unit weight of placenta, is about 2 per cent of that of lung. About 17 per cent of the oxygen supplied to the conceptus is utilized within the placenta to support such functions as active transport and hormone synthesis.

Gases cross the placenta by simple diffusion, and the process is therefore governed by Fick's law:

$$\frac{dm}{dt} = \frac{DA}{b}(C_1 - C_2)$$

where dm/dt = amount of gas transferred across placenta in unit time;

D = diffusion constant (i.e. diffusion coefficient multiplied by solubility of gas in water). For gases in solution the diffusion constant is thus directly proportional to solubility (which is some 30 times greater for carbon dioxide than for oxygen);

A = area of exchange;

b = thickness of placental membrane;

$C_1 - C_2$ = concentration gradient (expressed for gases as partial pressure differences between maternal and fetal blood).

Although blood oxygen saturation, content and partial pressure are all lower in the fetus than in the adult, the fetus normally has enough oxygen for all its metabolic needs and rarely needs to derive energy from anaerobic glycolysis. Fetuses can, however, survive periods of anoxia better than adult animals, a phenomenon also demonstrable in neonates.

Measurement of the partial pressures of respiratory gases in the fetus can be performed on blood samples collected via chronically implanted catheters in animals. In the human measurements can be made on umbilical cord blood samples collected during labour, but such measurements probably do not reflect partial pressures in the normal fetus. In Figure 6.2 two sets of data are provided for fetal and maternal blood gas partial pressures, one for human umbilical cord blood at parturition, and the other for the chronically catheterized sheep fetus. The latter may bear at least as much, if not more, resemblance to the normal human fetus in utero.

The transfer of oxygen from mother to fetus is influenced by:

The different oxygen dissociation curves of mother and fetus (Fig. 6.3a) If maternal and fetal blood are at the same temperature and pH, then the oxygen saturation curve for fetal blood lies to the left of that for maternal blood; the affinity of fetal blood for oxygen is thus greater. The main reason for this difference is the higher concentration of 2,3 diphosphoglycerate (DPG) in the erythrocytes of the adult, together with the lower binding capacity for DPG of

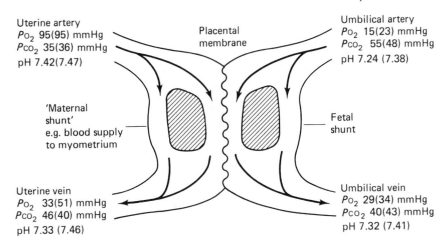

Uterine artery
Po_2 95(95) mmHg
Pco_2 35(36) mmHg
pH 7.42(7.47)

Placental
membrane

Umbilical artery
Po_2 15(23) mmHg
Pco_2 55(48) mmHg
pH 7.24 (7.38)

'Maternal
shunt'
e.g. blood supply
to myometrium

Fetal
shunt

Uterine vein
Po_2 33(51) mmHg
Pco_2 46(40) mmHg
pH 7.33 (7.46)

Umbilical vein
Po_2 29(34) mmHg
Pco_2 40(43) mmHg
pH 7.32 (7.41)

Fig. 6.2 A schematic representation of placental gas exchange. 'Shunts' represent blood flows that are not exposed to the placental membrane for exchange; on the maternal side this includes the blood which supplies the myometrium (about 20 per cent of uterine blood flow). Uterine and umbilical veins contain a mixture of blood from shunts and blood exposed to exchange at a membrane. The first of each pair of numbers is based on data gathered from the human at the time of birth; the numbers in brackets are based on data gathered in the chronically catheterized sheep fetus. The latter data may represent the situation *during* human pregnancy more accurately than the former. (Modified from Dancis, J. and Schneider, H. (1975). In: *The Placenta*. Ed. by P. Gruenwald. Medical and Technical Publishing Co. Ltd., Lancaster).

fetal haemoglobin (HbF), which has α and γ chains in its molecule, compared with that of adult haemoglobin (HbA), which has α and β chains. In particular, it is the γ chain which accounts for the reduced DPG binding by HbF. A reduction in DPG binding results in an increase in the oxygen affinity of the haemoglobin.

The different haemoglobin concentrations of mother and fetus (Fig. 6.3b) There is a higher concentration of haemoglobin in fetal blood than in maternal blood. (The magnitude of the difference is disputed; fetal stress can increase the fetal haematocrit, and umbilical cord blood samples collected perinatally may not be representative of the blood of the fetus in utero.) High fetal haemoglobin concentration results in an oxygen capacity greater than that of maternal blood, though this effect is partially offset by the fact that fetal haemoglobin, when fully saturated, carries less oxygen per gram (1.26 ml) than maternal haemoglobin (1.35 ml).

The 'Double Bohr effect' (Figs, 6.3 c and d) When fetal blood passes through the placenta it loses carbon dioxide and acidity, and consequently gains oxygen affinity; for maternal blood the changes are in the opposite direction. The combination of the two effects promote oxygen transfer from mother to fetus.

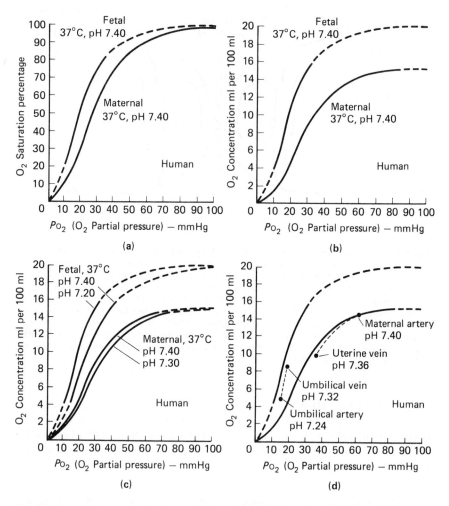

Fig. 6.3 Dissociation curves for human fetal and maternal blood samples taken during labour. Fetal arterial and venous samples probably contain less oxygen, more carbon dioxide, and more haemoglobin, and have a lower pH, than might be expected during undisturbed pregnancy. (a) Oxyhaemoglobin curves. Abcissa shows oxygen tension; ordinate expresses the percentage-saturation of haemoglobin with oxygen. (b) The same curves when the percentage-saturation values are converted to oxygen concentration; the difference between (a) and (b) is caused by the higher haemoglobin concentration in fetal blood. This effect may be exaggerated by the high haematocrit of fetal blood during labour. (c) The effect of pH on the dissociation curves. (d) Representative values reported for oxygen concentrations in blood samples from uterine and umbilical vessels placed on oxyhaemoglobin dissociation curves appropriate to the pH of each blood sample. During placental gas exchange, oxygen tension in maternal blood falls along the dotted line on the right, departing from the dissociation curve for pH 7.4 as the blood pH falls due to the influx of carbon dioxide and fixed acids from the fetal circulation. Reciprocal changes occur in fetal blood during its passage from the umbilical artery to the umbilical vein, the oxygen tension and concentration rising along the dotted line on the left. (From Metcalfe, J., Bartels, H. and Moll, W. (1967). *Physiological Reviews* **47**, 782–838).

Patterns of placental blood flow The direction of fetal and maternal blood flow relative to each other at the placental interface could in theory exert an influence on the efficiency of gaseous exchange. If the gases diffuse readily, then a countercurrent system of flow, with the two bloods flowing past each other in opposite directions, would have particular advantages. In the human, however, the predominant direction of maternal blood flow is probably at right angles to fetal blood flow — a 'crosscurrent' system; this is less effective than a countercurrent system, but more effective than a concurrent system (in which the flows are in the same direction) would be.

Fetal and maternal blood flow rates The slower the flow rates, the more complete the equilibration of partial pressures between the two bloods is likely to be, but, of course, the less the total amount of gas transfer between mother and fetus.

Placental diffusing capacity This is rarely a limiting factor to blood gas transfer unless it is reduced by degenerative changes in the placenta.

Maternal and fetal oxygen partial pressures Under normal circumstances these remain relatively stable. Values for PO_2 in human fetal blood obtained during the perinatal period, during which a degree of fetal hypoxia might be expected, may misrepresent the values in utero (see Fig. 6.2). At high altitude, maternal arterial PO_2 falls, and a compensatory increase in fetal erythropoiesis results. The mechanism by which erythropoiesis is regulated early in fetal life is not known, but by the third trimester (i.e. by the last three months of gestation) endogenous control by fetal erythropoietin is established.

Amount of carbon dioxide exchange Carbon dioxide is carried in the fetus in the same way as it is in the adult, i.e. approximately 62 per cent as bicarbonate, 30 per cent combined to haemoglobin as carbaminohaemoglobin, and 8 per cent in solution. The concentration of carbonic anhydrase is low in the fetal erythrocyte, but this does not appear to limit placental CO_2 exchange. Fetal blood has a lower affinity for CO_2 than maternal blood, and this affinity decreases as it gains oxygen; concurrently the opposite is happening in maternal blood, and this 'Christiansen–Douglas–Haldane effect' favours transfer of CO_2 from fetus to mother.

Water
Studies with labelled 'heavy' water indicate a very high level of water exchange occurring at an hourly rate of up to 3.5 litres. Net water flux is, of course, much lower. Water moves passively and very readily across the placenta in response to osmotic forces and if maternal osmotic pressure is raised by, say, an infusion of sucrose in the pregnant rabbit, a comparable rise in fetal plasma osmotic pressure occurs within 30 minutes. The net flux of water from the maternal to the fetal compartment during pregnancy is presumably the result of modest osmotic forces created by the synthesis of fetal macromolecules, and from the diffusion and transport of various electrolytes to the fetus.

Electrolytes

Electrolyte movement across the placenta can occur both by diffusion and by active transport. Diffusion will be influenced by gradients of both chemical concentration and electrical potential. In the sheep there is a transplacental potential difference such that the fetus is 50 mV negative with respect to the mother. In the human there is a negligible potential difference. Ions such as sodium, chloride and potassium, which are present in fairly equal concentrations in the blood of human mother and fetus, are thus believed to be exchanged largely by simple diffusion.

Exchange of sodium between human mother and fetus reaches its peak at about 35 weeks of pregnancy, and then falls rapidly. Sodium exchange is about 1000 times greater than the rate of fetal accumulation. The rapid reduction in sodium exchange towards the end of gestation may be regarded as evidence for a progressive inefficiency in placental exchange, and is possibly associated with the accumulation of fibrin deposits which cover about 8 per cent of placental villi at term.

Transport mechanisms from mother to fetus probably exist for iodide, calcium and iron which are present in fetal blood in higher concentrations than in maternal blood. In rabbits, iron transfer has been shown to involve extraction of iron by the placenta from the specific protein 'transferrin', to which iron is bound in plasma. The placenta concentrates a substantial amount of iron within itself.

Carbohydrate

Glucose is probably the most important metabolic fuel of the fetus. Its relatively high molecular weight and low lipid solubility would lead us to expect it to diffuse too slowly across the placenta to meet fetal need. The diffusion is, however, *facilitated* by the presence of a carrier molecule shuttling back and forth across the placental membrane to speed the rate of transfer without the expenditure of energy. The transfer system is specific for particular stereoisomers (D- rather than L-glucose) and for particular hexoses (glucose being transferred ten times faster than fructose). Glucose transfer in the human placenta is very rapid, and maternal concentration is consistently higher than fetal so that net transfer to the fetus is always 'downhill'.

Amino acids

Amino acids are utilized by the fetus both for protein synthesis and for energy requirements. Most amino acids appear to be transported by stereospecific active transport mechanisms; thus fetal plasma levels of most amino acids are higher than maternal levels with concentration ratios ranging from 6 : 5 to 4 : 1. The transport mechanisms are saturable, and inhibition may occur when two amino acids are being transported at high rates — indicating competition for transfer sites. An exception to transfer by active transport is cystine, which is present in lower concentration in fetal than in maternal plasma, indicating that facilitated diffusion may well be involved.

Protein

Protein transfer does occur across the human placenta in spite of its large

Table 6.1 The relative levels of some constituents in maternal and fetal cord blood, with a note on their placental transfer mechanism

	About equal	Lower in fetus	Higher in fetus	Transfer mechanism
Amino acids			+	Active transport
Urea	+			Diffusion
Uric acid	+			Diffusion
Creatinine	+			Diffusion
Inorganic phosphorus			+	Not known
Free fatty acids		+		Diffusion; some arise in placenta
Cholesterol		+		Diffusion; can arise in placenta
Glucose		+		Facilitated diffusion
Lactic acid			+	May arise in placenta
Calcium			+	Active transport
Magnesium	+			Diffusion + / − active transport
Chloride	+			Diffusion + / − active transport
Sodium	+			Diffusion + / − active transport
Potassium	+			Diffusion + / − active transport
Iron			+	Active transport
Vitamins				
Fat-soluble		+		Diffusion
Water-soluble			+	Active transport
hCG		+		Arises in placenta
hPL		+		Arises in placenta

molecular size. Transfer is at a lower rate than for amino acids and probably occurs by pinocytosis involving uptake by specific receptors on the placental surface. In the human γ-*globulins* of the IgG groups are transferred at twice the rate of albumins, even though their molecular weight is twice as great — a process which increases in efficiency towards term. The consequence of this transfer is that the fetus is born with IgG levels similar to those of the mother. The placental transfer of *albumins* is probably sufficient to provide a significant amount of fetal plasma albumin, but the fetal liver can synthesize albumin quite early in gestation so the fetus does not depend entirely on maternal supplies. Polypeptide hormones and thyroxine probably cross the placenta too slowly to influence the normal fetus, which matures early and functions autonomously so far as these hormones are concerned (but see p. 118).

Lipids
Lipid-soluble molecules generally cross the placenta easily unless bound to proteins, or conjugated as sulphates or glucuronides, which renders them polar, water-soluble and relatively impermeant.

Free fatty acids (FFAs) circulate in plasma bound to albumin. They are transported early in pregnancy at a rate which keeps pace with the rate of fetal fat synthesis, but the rapid fat deposition in the third trimester exceeds the capacity for placental FFA transfer, and must mainly arise by *de novo* synthesis in the fetus. Phospholipids and cholesterol, being transported in the lipoprotein fraction in plasma, are very slowly transferred. Unconjugated steroids such as oestrogens, progesterone and testosterone are probably readily transported in both directions across the placenta, but polar conjugates (sulphates and glucuronides) are transferred very slowly; in the case of sulphates there are placental sulphatases which may facilitate transfer. All three oestrogens (oestradiol, oestrone and oestriol) are present in fetal blood at about ten times the concentration found in maternal blood, yet little if any of these oestrogens originates from fetal tissues.

Vitamins
Vitamin transfer occurs readily for the fat-soluble vitamins (A, D, E and K). Vitamin A is probably transferred as the pro-vitamin carotene, being converted within the fetus to vitamin A (retinol). Stores of vitamin K are very limited in the newborn, and it is given to all newborn babies to prevent the deficiency which can result in defective blood clotting. The water-soluble vitamins (C, B_1, B_2, B_6, B_{12}, folic and folinic acid) are generally present in fetal blood in higher concentrations than in maternal blood, suggesting the existence of active transport mechanisms in the placenta.

Waste products
Waste product transfer encompasses movement of CO_2, urea, uric acid, creatinine and bilirubin. Bilirubin is considered on pp. 109–110. Urea levels in the fetus are normally higher than those in the mother, and the placenta is permeable to urea which therefore diffuses down a concentration gradient. Some 40 per cent of the nitrogen entering the fetus as amino acids is returned to the mother as urea.

Drugs (Steele: Gynaecology, Obstetrics and the Neonate, Chapter 11)
Drug transfer occurs quite readily in the case of lipid-soluble drugs such as local and general anaesthetics, and alcohol, all of which may depress the function of the fetal central nervous system. Withdrawal symptoms may arise in newborn babies born to habitual users of barbiturates or opiates, indicating that they must reach the fetus from the mother. Certain antibacterial drugs may cross, though some penicillins are retarded by plasma binding. Drugs which are in use and are known to have harmful effects include *streptomycin*, which can damage the fetal auditory nerve, and *sulphonamides*, which, although they do not readily cross the placenta, may displace bilirubin from its plasma binding sites; the bilirubin thereby freed may then cause brain damage in the neonate.

Other placental functions

As well as acting as the interface for exchange between mother and fetus, there are other important placental functions.

The placenta as an endocrine gland
The production of protein hormones by the placenta is considered on pp. 83–85, and its production of steroid hormones is described on pp. 119–122. Their role in the control of parturition, lactation and maternal behaviour is discussed in Chapters 8 and 9, and a systematic description of the major placental hormones is given in Chapter 10.

The placenta as an immunological barrier
This function is discussed later in this Chapter (see pp. 89–90).

The physiology of the pregnant mother

The fetus is an egoist, not merely a helpless dependent. Its purpose is to see that its own needs are served, and this is achieved by causing a substantial upheaval to its mother's physiology. The changes in maternal physiology serve to ensure maternal well-being, and to ensure that the fetal 'supply-line' works effectively. Futhermore, in the post-partum period, the mother must be able to provide the neonate with the requisite care to ensure its nutrition, resistance to infection, thermoregulation and psychological development (Steele: *Gynaecology, Obstetrics and the Neonate*, Chapter 1).

Maternal endocrinology

Ovarian and placental hormones (Fig. 6.4)
Of all the changes in maternal physiology which occur during pregnancy, the most characteristic are hormonal. The earliest symptom of human pregnancy is amenorrhoea which arises because the corpus luteum, formed in the ovary after ovulation, does not undergo lysis at the end of a two-week lifespan (as would be the case if there were no pregnancy), but is maintained. The maintenance of the corpus luteum ensures that there is a continued supply of ovarian progesterone which is needed to prevent degenerative changes in the endometrium that lead, in primates, to menstruation. In non-primate mammals, the maintenance of the corpus luteum may be due either to the presence of prolactin (e.g. in the rat) or to the failure of the pregnant uterus to produce a luteolytic substance (believed to be prostaglandin $F_{2\alpha}$) which, when released by the non-pregnant uterus, acts on the ovary to cause lysis of the corpus luteum. Evidence for the latter mechanism includes the failure of the corpus luteum of the sheep to undergo lysis at the expected time after ovulation if the uterus has been removed. In contrast, hysterectomy in primates does not prevent lysis of the corpus luteum.

What controls the lifespan of the human corpus luteum? In the woman, implantation of the fertilized blastocyst occurs just six days after ovulation, and from about this time a luteotrophic hormone — human chorionic gonadotrophin (hCG) — is produced. This hormone can be detected in maternal peripheral blood shortly after implantation, well before the time when the corpus luteum normally regresses in non-pregnant women. It therefore seems reasonable to suppose that the corpus luteum is maintained by hCG produced by the developing conceptus; immunization against this hormone has been shown to block pregnancy in several species of primates. Human chorionic gonadotrophin has been detected in the blood of women fitted with intrauterine contraceptive devices; this finding indicates that these devices may be incorrectly named since the hCG in these women is presumably secreted by trophoblast tissue resulting from conception.

The placenta is the source of a second protein hormone which first appears in maternal plasma during the sixth to eighth week of pregnancy. This

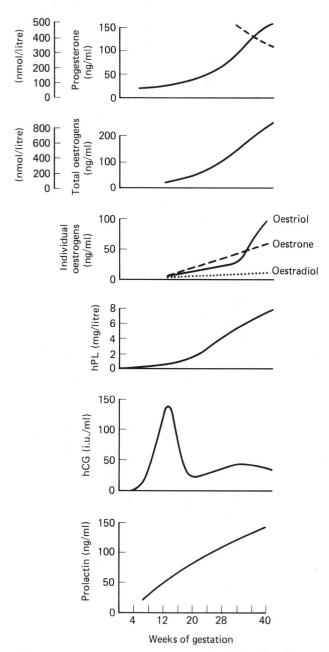

Fig. 6.4 'Typical' values for the concentration of certain hormones in maternal plasma during pregnancy. The presence of both a solid line and a dotted line in the graph at the top of the figure indicates the uncertainty in the current literature as to whether or not progesterone levels fall prior to parturition; it will persist until discrepancies between assay methods have been resolved.

hormone — human placental lactogen (hPL) — sometimes known as chorionic somatomammotrophin (hCS) — is secreted by the syncytiotrophoblast cells of the placental villi at a rate which rises to at least one gram per day. In spite of its name, the effects of hPL on breast development are relatively weak compared with those of prolactin. It also has growth hormone-like actions, promoting lipolysis and a rise in plasma levels of triglycerides and free fatty acids. Human placental lactogen inhibits the action of insulin on glucose utilization, but enhances the incorporation of amino acids into protein. The overall effect is to conserve maternal glucose thereby making more available to the fetus. The effects of hPL are broadly 'anti-insulin', accounting in part for the decreased glucose tolerance which occurs during pregnancy, and explaining the need for pregnant diabetic mothers to increase their insulin dosage. An additional function of both hCG and hPL may be to act as consituents of the surface layer of glycoprotein which could protect syncytiotrophoblast cells from immunological attack by the mother (see p. 90).

The existence of hCG and hPL has been known for more than 50 and 20 years respectively. More recently at least four other proteins have been isolated from the plasma of pregnant women and from the placenta. These include *human chorionic thyrotrophin* and a β-globulin known as PSβ$_2$G. Pregnancy is terminated in monkeys injected with antibodies to the latter hormone, suggesting that it may be concerned in the prevention of maternal rejection of the fetus.

Shortly after the onset of protein hormone secretion, the placenta develops the capacity for synthesizing and secreting steroid hormones. Initially it produces progesterone, and subsequently oestriol is produced in large quantities, together with smaller amounts of other steroids. Since the steroidogenic activities of the placenta are intimately related to fetal adrenal cortical function, detailed consideration of this topic will be postponed (see pp. 119–122).

Other changes in maternal hormones

The adenohypophysis increases in size during pregnancy. Prolactin arises from acidophilic cells known as *lactotrophs*, which account for 0.5 per cent of the total number of adenohypophysial cells in the nonpregnant woman, but for 18 per cent or more during pregnancy. The amount of prolactin within the maternal pituitary gland increases from about the eighth week of pregnancy and its concentration in maternal plasma rises throughout pregnancy. Prolactin exerts lactogenic effects when progesterone levels fall after parturition, but it has no known role during human pregnancy.

Maternal insulin levels are raised in pregnancy during the fasting state and after a glucose load; the increased insulin secretion may strain pancreatic reserves. The half-life of insulin is reduced. Maternal concentrations of adrenal steroids rise during pregnancy mainly as the result of a rise in cortisol-binding-globulin (CBG) concentrations; since bound cortisol is inactive, the rise in cortisol levels during pregnancy produces no obvious effects. The rise in CBG concentration is thought to result from an increase in the synthesis of the globulin by the maternal liver stimulated by oestrogens secreted in increasing quantities by the placenta. Aldosterone concentration is highest in the first three months of pregnancy, then falls progressively.

Other changes in maternal physiology

Table 6.2 lists some alterations in maternal physiology occurring during a typical human pregnancy involving a single human fetus. Changes occurring in twin pregnancies are normally less than twice as large.

Table 6.2 Some typical values of various parameters in nonpregnant women, and in women in late pregnancy

	'Typical' nonpregnant	'Typical' pregnant
Total body weight	65 kg	77.5 kg
Total body water	39 litre	46 litre*
Blood volume	4.2 litre	5.8 litre
Plasma volume	2.75 litre	4.0 litre
Red cell volume	1.4 litre	1.8 litre
Oxygen uptake at rest	250 ml/min	300 ml/min
Cardiac output	5 litre/min	6.5 litre/min
Stroke volume	70 ml	87 ml
Heart rate	72 /min	87 /min
Renal blood flow	900 ml/min	1000 ml/min**
Plasma cortisol-binding globulin	30 ng/litre	70 ng/litre

*Of which 2.3 litres in fetus; 2.1 litres in placenta, uterus and amniotic fluid; 1.25 litres in maternal plasma; 1.35 litres caused by maternal tissue fluid retention.

**But rises to 1200 ml/min during second trimester.

Cardiovascular system

Plasma protein concentration falls and total red cell volume rises, but not enough to prevent a reduction in haematocrit caused by plasma volume expansion. The reduction in plasma protein concentration will influence the 'Starling forces' at work in the formation and reabsorption of interstitial fluid by capillaries, and will contribute to the increase in tissue fluid volume which may result in visible oedema. Fibrinogen levels increase during pregnancy with a consequent elevation of erythrocyte sedimentation rate. The rise in cardiac output may not be present in late pregnancy if the pregnant woman lies on her back, causing abdominal contents to obstruct return of blood via the inferior vena cava; this can lead to faintness ('supine hypotension syndrome') which disappears when the woman lies on her side.

Elevation of the diaphragm displaces the heart into a more transverse position during pregnancy. Mean arterial blood pressure is normally unaltered because the rise in cardiac output is offset by a fall in peripheral resistance attributable largely to the fact that the placenta serves as a low-resistance arteriovenous shunt. Pulse pressure measured at the brachial artery increases somewhat. A modest rise in mean arterial pressure is not, however, uncommon; a rise to hypertensive levels (about 140/90 mmHg systolic/diastolic) coupled with visible oedema and the presence of albumin in the urine constitutes the pathological condition of *pre-eclampsia* (Steele: *Gynaecology, Obstetrics and the Neonate,* Chapter 10). Venous pressure in the legs increases progressively during pregnancy owing to compression of the pelvic veins and the inferior vena cava by the uterus, but arm and central venous pressures do not rise.

The respiratory system

The pregnant woman is affected by upward pressure on the diaphragm as the uterus enlarges, though the resulting sense of breathlessness commonly decreases when the fetal head descends into the pelvis. A second respiratory effect — increased oxygen consumption and carbon dioxide exhalation — arises from the increase in the amount of metabolically active tissue which causes an increase in oxygen uptake of about 15 per cent in late pregnancy compared with basal uptake in the nonpregnant state.

Renal function

There is a reduction in the tubular maximum reabsorptive capacity for glucose which may contribute to glycosuria. Levels of amino acids, particularly histidine, may rise in the urine due to increased filtration and decreased reabsorption. Bladder function is affected particularly during the early stages of pregnancy when the enlarging uterus is resting on the bladder within the pelvic cavity; there results an increase in the frequency of micturition.

Maternal metabolism

Profound changes occur in maternal carbohydrate and fat metabolism during pregnancy. There is a shift towards the metabolism of fat in peripheral maternal tissues which ensure that sufficient glucose is available for the metabolic demands of the maternal brain and the conceptus. Blood levels of lactate, pyruvate, phospholipids and free fatty acids rise, but fasting blood glucose level does not. The causes of the observed changes are poorly understood; alteration in hPL and, to a lesser extent, insulin levels are undoubtedly important, but metabolic effects of oestrogens and progesterone cannot be discounted.

The skin

There is an increase in cutaneous blood flow during pregnancy. Skin pigmentation tends to darken probably as a result of elevated levels of melanocyte stimulating hormone. 'Stretch marks' (*striae gravidarum*) may develop in the skin of the abdomen, breasts and hips in the latter months of pregnancy. Scalp, facial and body hair may increase in thickness during pregnancy.

Mammary glands

The changes occurring in the mammary glands during pregnancy are discussed in Chapter 9.

The mouth and gut
There is an increase in vascularity of the gums; minor bleeding may result. Inflammation of the gums (*gingivitis*) is common, and teeth may loosen. The lower oesophageal sphincter may be displaced into the thorax and this, together with delayed gastric emptying which is seen during pregnancy, may predispose to increased reflux of gastric contents — causing 'heartburn'. Intestinal motility decreases, and there may be an increase in water and electrolyte reabsorption from the large intestine. These two factors may lead to constipation, which will exacerbate the tendency for the development of haemorrhoids which are associated with the pelvic hyperaemia seen in pregnancy.

Body weight (Fig. 6.5)
Women gain weight during pregnancy, but it is difficult to establish a normal value for this weight increase. It may range between 7 and 17 kg, with the average being about 11.5 kg. The distribution of the weight gain is shown in Fig. 6.5. Water accounts for more than half of the normal maternal weight gain during pregnancy, and total body water increases by about 7 litres by the 40th week of pregnancy, of which about 2.3 litres are within the fetus, about 1.4 litres are due to maternal tissue fluid retention, excluding fluid in placenta, uterus and amniotic cavity which accounts for about 2.1 litres.

Fat storage is common during pregnancy though the extent to which it is 'normal' is unclear. Well-nourished rats deposit fat in their bodies during

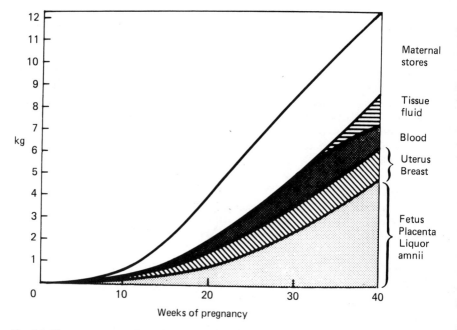

Fig. 6.5 The components of weight gain in normal pregnancy. (From Hytten, F.E. and Leitch, I. (1971). *The Physiology of Human Pregnancy*, 2nd edn. Blackwell, Oxford.)

pregnancy and lose this extra fat, and more, during lactation. For the human a readjustment of appetite during pregnancy to provide some caloric excess, which is laid down as fat, would appear to be biologically appropriate to provide a reserve of energy with which to produce breast milk. Women who do not breast feed after pregnancy must therefore restrict their diets if they are to lose the fat laid down during pregnancy.

The uterus
The uterus increases twenty-fold in weight during pregnancy. The size of the uterine cavity enlarges from a triangular potential space about 3 × 5 cm to contain 4.5–5 litres at term — or even more in multiple pregnancies. Uterine enlargement is caused by a combination of hyperplasia, hypertrophy, and stretching, and accounts for about 5 per cent of the total nitrogen retention during human pregnancy. The stimuli for this growth are both endocrine and mechanical. Oestrogens stimulate protein synthesis, an increase in water content, and some increase in the mitotic activity of uterine cells; the addition of progesterone greatly enhances mitosis. The striking changes in uterine blood flow occurring during pregnancy have already been mentioned.

Other changes in the endometrium and the myometrium associated with pregnancy either have been (p. 70) or will be (pp. 132–133) described elsewhere, and the specific effects of oestrogens, progestagens and prostaglandins on the uterus are described in Chapter 10.

Central nervous system
Apart from an increase in appetite there are no consistent behavioural or neurophysiological changes in human pregnancy. A culturally-induced susceptibility to the blandishments of persons selling baby care equipment, necessary and unnecessary, is to be expected. Emotional instability is quite common, women tend to be more easily fatigued, and they experience anxiety about their impending parturition and about the health of their unborn child. Cravings for particular foods, and pica (appetite for bizarre materials such as coal or soap) are sometimes reported. Nausea and vomiting ('morning sickness') may be seen during the sixth to the twelfth week of pregnancy, and backache may be reported in the later stages. Certain animals show a crescendo of nest-building activity as parturition approaches — a behaviour which can be intitiated in virgin animals by appropriate hormone treatment.

Immunological considerations in pregnancy and thereafter

Why does the mother not immunologically reject the fetus?

The fetus inherits cell-surface histocompatibility antigens from both parents. Those inherited from the father will be foreign to the mother and the fetus can thus be regarded as an allograft. The mother is not immunologically incompetent: antibodies to fetal antigens can be detected in the maternal circulation, and grafting of fetal tissues results in their rejection. If a mother is actively immunized against paternal antigens, she can still establish and maintain a pregnancy by that father. The earliest contact with foreign antigens in the reproductive process is at sexual intercourse, when spermatozoa, bearing antigens, are deposited in the female tract. Sensitization rarely occurs, probably because too few spermatozoa pass the cervix to be immunogenic, but it could be a rare cause of infertility.

Perhaps the mother, in spite of her immunological competence, is somehow specifically desensitized to antigens derived from the father? Studies with skin grafts provide no evidence for this. Nor is there any reason to believe that the uterus is an 'immunologically privileged site', i.e. an area where allografts can survive without immunological attack; allografts of most tissues in the uterus (e.g. parathyroid gland) are rejected in the normal way.

Is there any evidence for *local* effects resulting from high concentrations of steroid hormones produced by trophoblast cells? Apparently not, because transplanted trophoblast will not protect adjacent allografts of other tissues from rejection. The most plausible explanation for the survival of the fetal allograft is that a *barrier* separates fetal and maternal cells. In the haemochorial human placenta, trophoblast is in direct contact with maternal blood. The maternal surface of the trophoblast must therefore be the site of the frontier between fetus and mother; either this surface lacks histocompatibility antigens, or more probably, these antigens are masked by a surface layer of glycoprotein which prevents them from eliciting an immune response from the maternal tissues. The barrier must be imperfect, for some maternal immune reaction to fetal antigen is common. Placental glycoprotein (e.g. hCG) and polypeptide (e.g. hPL) hormones may contribute to the barrier: they are present in quantity, can exert immunosuppressive effects, and are localized in the glycoprotein coat secreted by, and adherent to, syncytiotrophoblast.

The development of immune mechanisms in the fetus and neonate

Immune responses are due either to blood-borne antibodies (antibody-mediated immunity) or to cells (cell-mediated immunity). Both depend on the activity of small lymphocytes which differentiate to form two distinct populations, one thymus-derived (*T lymphocytes* or *T cells*) and the other bone-marrow-derived (*B lymphocytes* or *B cells*). T lymphocytes are found mainly in the deep cortical areas of the lymph nodes and account for about 80 per cent of the circulating lymphocytes. B lymphocytes originate mainly in the bone marrow, and possibly also in gut-associated lymphoid tissues such as the appendix and Peyer's patches. They are less mobile than T cells, being found in, for example, peripheral lymphoid organs and lymph nodes. They account for about 20 per cent of the lymphocytes in the peripheral blood. B cells differentiate under antigenic stimulation into plasma cells which are responsible for the synthesis and secretion of all forms of antibody and all circulating immunoglobulins (Igs). B cells are distinguishable by the presence of immunoglobulin (Ig) bound to their surface, and normally only one class of Ig is found on any B lymphocyte. B lymphocytes bearing membrane-bound Ig are first found in the liver of human fetuses in the 10th week of development, and in the spleen during the 12th week.

The immunoglobulins
The humoral antibodies are the immunoglobulins, i.e. serum globulins the main property of which is their antibody actvity. They are divided into five classes designated IgG, IgA, IgM, IgD and IgE, according to their distinctive heavy polypeptide chains.

IgG globulins IgG globulins account for 70–80 per cent of all Ig in adult serum, and are synthesized in plasma cells in spleen, lymph nodes and the lamina propria (but not the mucosa) of the intestine. IgG is normally produced only in trace amounts by the fetus, full synthesis of IgG beginning at weeks 3–4 after birth. Immunization in adults results in the appearance of the appropriate IgG antibody in the serum, but in the newborn infant it may be ineffective because maternally-derived antibodies tend to neutralize the antigen before it can elicit antibody formation in the infant. IgG neutralizes bacteria and/or bacterial toxins, and viruses. It is the only Ig that is actively transferred in significant amounts through the placenta from mother to fetus, there being a site on the IgG molecule which permits active transfer through the placenta. IgG has the longest half-life (about 33 days in the newborn and 17 days in the adult).

IgA globulins IgA globulins comprise about 10–15 per cent of the Ig in the normal adult, and they are the principal secretory form of antibody. Like IgG, IgA is produced by plasma cell derivatives, and much of it is secreted actively into colostrum and milk, tears, respiratory system and gastrointestinal tract, by acinar and epithelial cells of the mucosal surfaces. There are structural differences between IgA molecules depending on whether the IgA is obtained from secretions or from serum; *secretory IgA* is a polymer composed of two identical monomeric molecules coupled by a unique peptide synthesized in epithelial cells.

In normal adults, IgA-producing cells are most abundant in mucosa of the intestine, and are also found next to glandular structures of the body such as the nasal mucosa. These local IgA-producing cells develop very soon after birth, and IgA is detectable in saliva of newborn babies before it can be detected in serum. *Serum IgA* is unable to pass *from* serum *to* the exocrine gland, though much of the serum IgA arises from plasma cells in the exocrine glands and therefore shares the same antibody specificities as secretory IgA.

IgA is not produced by the normal fetus, and it passes from mother to fetus in minimal amounts. IgA synthesis begins 2 to 4 weeks after birth, and it has a half-life of 6 days. Thus if the mucosal surfaces of the neonate are to be adequately coated with IgA, it must come from the mother's breast milk, into which it is secreted in large quantities.

Other immunoglobulins IgM globulins comprise between 5 and 10 per cent of the total serum Ig. Unlike IgG globulins they are mainly confined to the circulation and do not migrate into extravascular spaces. IgM globulins are synthesized in certain plasma cells, and in reticular cells of the spleen and lymph nodes. They are normally produced in only small amounts by the fetus, though they are produced in large quantities in the presence of intrauterine infection, resulting in the presence of high levels at birth. IgM is the first class of globulin to appear after immunization, and it is the predominant class produced by neonates in response to antigen challenge. IgM synthesis increases rapidly within 2 to 5 days of birth. It has a half-life of 5 days and does not cross the human placenta.

IgE globulins have a particular role in allergic reactions; they do not cross the placenta, so that babies rarely exhibit their mother's allergies.

Immunoglobulins in maternal blood
Albumin concentrations are reduced, but concentrations of globulins are unchanged or slightly increased. There is evidence in about 5 per cent of pregnant women for maternal immunization by components of the fetal blood, including HLA antigens and both rhesus and other red blood cell antigens; the frequency of antibody detection in mothers increases in subsequent pregnancies.

Immunoglobulins in fetal and neonatal blood (Fig 6.6)
Blood levels of IgG increase from about the 13th week of gestation, and fetal levels equal maternal levels by the 34th week. Ig globulins are found in only small amounts in normal fetuses, and IgA, IgD and IgE are present in small amounts, if at all. The fetus and newborn are no longer regarded as immuno-logically incompetent; the fetal spleen can synthesize IgG and IgM to some extent from the 20th week of gestation, but not IgA or IgD. The placenta is probably not a site of immunoglobulin production. Most of the IgG in the fetus is provided by the mother. There is a close correlation between the absolute concentration of γ-globulins, in particular IgG, in the mother and the fetus. In mice transfer of IgG from mother to fetus appears to involve two processes: one of these exhibits first-order kinetics and is presumably diffusion, while the other is a carrier or enzymatic process which is active, specific for IgG, and is inhibited by very high maternal IgG concentrations. Thus the placenta is a rare example of a non-endodermal membrane selectively permeable to proteins; IgG is apparently taken up by the human syncytiotrophoblast by pinocytosis and escapes to the opposite side into the intervillous space of the placental villi.

Although IgG antibodies attain similar levels on both sides of the placenta, antibodies belonging to the IgA or IgM class are either absent or much less concentrated in cord blood than in maternal blood. In the case of many widespread and highly contagious diseases, antibodies can be found in almost all adults, and since the antibodies are of the IgG class, the offspring are protected for the first few months after birth. In the case of rare diseases, or those in which the persistence of antibodies is shorter in the adult, such as plague and cholera, newborn babies may be unprotected. In spite of their fairly short half-life maternal antibodies can be detected in the child for 6–9 months after birth.

The ease of transfer of maternal antibodies may be related to placental structure, and disappearance of uterine epithelium from the placenta may

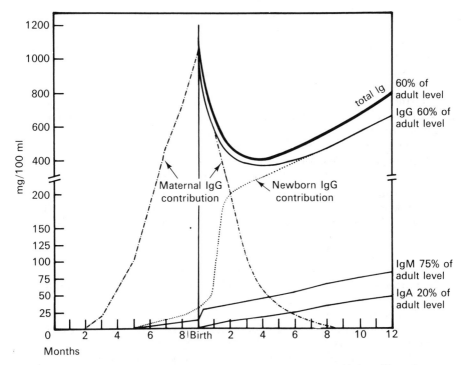

Fig. 6.6 Total Ig and IgG, IgA, and IgM levels in the human fetus and infant. (From De Muralt, G. (1978). In: *Perinatal Physiology.* Ed. by U. Stave. Plenum, New York.)

contribute to its permeability to maternal IgG. In cows, goats, sheep and horses, in which the uterine epithelium is not eroded, the newborn are without detectable γ globulins, but in such animals these substances are transferred for about 36 hours after birth via colostrum and milk and absorbed by the gut.

In the postnatal period, γ-globulin levels decline over the first 3 months. The decline is due to:

1. The catabolism of maternal γ-globulins.
2. Some loss due to secretion into the intestinal tract.
3. Insufficient synthesis by the neonate.
4. Dilution of the transmitted IgG in an expanding volume of plasma and tissue fluids.

Near-adult values of the IgG are not attained until about 12–18 months of age. IgA levels at birth are very low, but detectable at 6 weeks; they reach adult values by 12–16 years. IgM values are low at birth, then rise very rapidly to reach about half the adult level by 3 to 6 months. This postnatal pattern of immunoglobulin level is influenced by:

1. The length of pregnancy, both γ-globulin and IgG levels being lower in premature babies.

2. Birth weight, IgG levels being low in small-for-dates newborn babies (see p. 96).

3. Nutritional state: a reduced intake of dietary protein reduces the production of immunoglobulins.

4. Naturally occuring infections in the fetus, some of which can promote antibody production by the fetus.

5. Inoculation with antigens: postnatal inoculation can stimulate antibody formation even in very small babies. If maternal antibodies have entered the infant either via the placenta (IgG) or via the colostrum (IgA) the antigens introduced into the baby do not promote antibody production as effectively as in infants lacking maternal antibody.

6. Effect of immunoglobins absorbed from colostrum and milk.

The antibodies which pass from a mother to her baby include not only desirable antibodies against invading pathogens, but may occasionally include antigens involved in auto-immune reactions; newborn tissues which may be affected by such antibodies include thyroid, neuromuscular junction and heart.

Breast milk: its importance in transfer of surface antibodies
Colostrum and milk represent an abundant source of IgM and, especially, of IgA. There is a high milk : serum IgA ratio, which is evidence for local production within the mammary gland. The IgA consumption of a breast-fed infant is maintained at a steady level over the first four months of lactation. The secretory IgA molecule is highly resistant to the pH changes and proteolytic enzymes found in the gut. IgG is actively and specifically transported into human milk, and IgM is also transmitted through the mammary glandular epithelium into milk.

The secretory IgA fraction includes antibodies against *Escherichia coli* (one of the most important neonatal pathogens), staphylococci, pneumococci, and polio virus. Although virtually none of the large supplies of immunoglobulin in human colostrum and milk are absorbed into the infant's circulation, breast-fed infants have better resistance than bottle-fed infants against many bacterial and viral infections; this is now attributed, at least in part, to the presence of secretory IgA in breast milk which exerts an important immune function at epithelial surfaces, particularly in the intestine where the bacterial and viral antibodies in the IgA protect against bacterial invasion and antigen uptake (Steele: *Gynaecology, Obstetrics and the Neonate*, Chapter 3).

Immunization, immune tolerance, and immune paralysis
The reaction of the neonate to antigens frequently involves antibody production, i.e. the development of immunity. Sometimes, however, a temporary (*immunological tolerance*) or permanent (*immunological paralysis*) incapacity to mount an immune response may be seen. The factors determining exactly how an infant will respond to an antigen exposure are complex, imperfectly understood, and unpredictable.

Further reading

Assali, N.S. and Brinkman, C.R. (eds)(1972). *Pathophysiology of Gestation. Vol. 1: Maternal Disorders*. Academic Press, New York.

Cauchi, M.N. (1981). *Obstetric and Perinatal Immunology.* Current Topics in Immunology Series. Edward Arnold, London.

Chamberlain, G. and Wilkinson, A. (eds)(1979). *Placental Transfer.* Pitman Medical, Tunbridge Wells.

Faber, J.J. and Thornberg, K.L. (eds)(1983). *Placental Physiology: Structure and Function of Fetomaternal Exchange.* Raven Press, New York.

Fuchs, F. and Klopper, A. (eds) (1971). *Endocrinology of Pregnancy*, 2nd edn. Harper and Row, Hagerstown, Maryland.

Gruenwald, P. (ed)(1975). *The Placenta.* MTP, Lancaster.

Hemmings, W.A. (ed)(1976). *Maternofoetal Transmission of Immunoglobulins.* Cambridge University Press, Cambridge.

Hogarth, P.J. (1982). *Immunological Aspects of Mammalian Reproduction.* Blackie, London.

Hytten, F.E. and Leitch, I. (1971). *The Physiology of Human Pregnancy*, 2nd edn. Blackwell Scientific, Oxford.

7

The fetus and neonate

Introduction

The fetus is thought of nowadays not as an inert passenger in pregnancy but, rather, as in command of it. The fetus, in collaboration with the placenta, (a) ensures the endocrine success of pregnancy, (b) induces changes in maternal physiology which make her a suitable host, (c) is responsible for solving the immunological problems which are raised by its intimate contact with its mother, and (d) determines the duration of pregnancy.

In this chapter a number of physiological systems will be followed from the fetal through the perinatal to the neonatal period. During fetal life, regulatory mechanisms must be established to ensure fetal autonomy and homeostasis, and must be in a state of readiness, at the end of gestation, to ensure neonatal survival.

Growth

Growth is perhaps the most obvious sign of fetal well-being, and lack of growth is a clear sign that all is not well (Steele: *Gynaecology, Obstetrics and the Neonate*, Chapter 5). The term 'growth' can have different meanings e.g. weight gain, head enlargement, length increase, and organ differentiation; weight gain is the most commonly used criterion. Babies weighing less than 2500 g at birth are defined by the term *low birth weight*. Low birth weight may occur (a) because a baby is born *preterm*, i.e. after too short a pregnancy or (b) because a baby is *small for dates* (SFD), i.e. the baby is more than two standard deviations below the weight expected for a baby of its post-conception age. About 30 per cent of low-birth-weight babies are full-term i.e. are of the normal post-conception age, and are therefore SFD.

Fetal growth up to the 10th week of pregnancy is relatively slow, expressed as weight gain per unit time (Fig. 7.1). The major fetal organ systems differentiate during that time, and subsequent development involves a large increase in mass. *Rate* of growth is maximal between the 28th and 36th week, and then falls. Growth rate expressed *incrementally* falls from about 6 per cent per day during the first 12 weeks and falls unsteadily to 1.3 per cent per day by the 38th week.

Protein accumulation occurs early in fetal development, reaching 300 g by

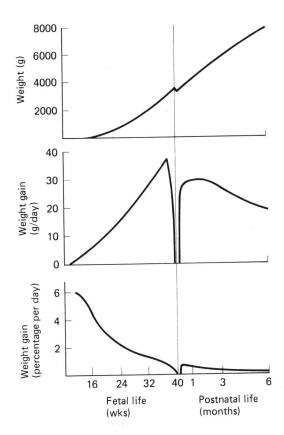

Fig. 7.1 Graphs showing average fetal and postnatal growth: (a) as absolute weight in grams (b) as growth rate in grams per day, and (c) as incremental growth rate i.e. percentage increase in body weight per day between the eighth week of fetal life and 6 months of postnatal life.

the 35th week; fat is deposited slowly at first but exceeds the weight of protein by the 38th week, and by term three times as much energy is stored as fat compared with that stored as protein. Ninety-five per cent of body mass of the young fetus is water, but this falls to 70 per cent by term; the ratio of extracellular to intracellular water is 4 : 1 at the 10th week and 1 : 1 at term.

The fetus is not the only component of uterine contents which enlarges during pregnancy (Fig. 7.2). Amniotic fluid increases in volume until the 34th week, and then declines. The rate of growth of the placenta is high early in pregnancy, then falls sharply. The result is a sharp reduction of the ratio of placental size: fetal size towards term, with the result that the placenta may become a limiting factor in fetal growth.

The factors which affect fetal growth may be divided into *fetal*, *placental* and *maternal*.

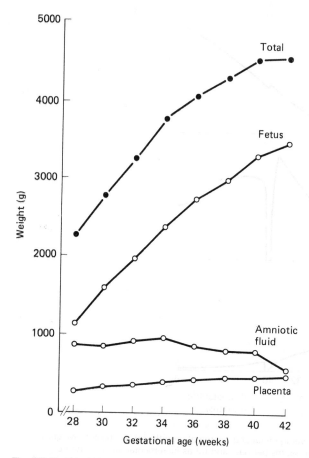

Fig. 7.2 Total weight of human conceptus and weights of fetus, amniotic fluid, and placenta from the 28th week of gestation. (From Biggers, J.D. (1980). In: *Medical Physiology*, vol. 2, 14th edn. Ed. by V.B. Mountcastle. C.V. Mosby, St Louis.)

Fetal factors

Genetic constitution
There are racial differences in mean birth weight even with optimal maternal nutrition, e.g. North American Indians 3.6 kg; Europeans 3.2 kg; Indians 2.9 kg. This may be due to inherent differences in the capacity of fetuses of different races to grow in utero, but may also be due to differences (either inherited or acquired during development) between mothers of different races in their capacity to provide for growth.

Damage to the fetus
Infections or teratogens retard growth not only of a specifically affected organ system, but also overall.

The sex of the fetus
Male neonates tend to be larger than females.

Fetal endocrine activity
A variety of fetal endocrine glands have been shown to be involved in the control of fetal growth in different species e.g. anterior pituitary, thyroid, parathyroid, pancreas and kidneys. In the human, the fetal pancreas clearly affects growth: maternal hyperglycaemia causes fetal hyperglycaemia which may stimulate insulin secretion from the fetal pancreas resulting in increased fetal growth. Thus mothers with poorly controlled diabetes have unusually large babies. The fetal thyroid seems to be dispensable for normal human prenatal growth, and hypothyroid neonates may even be slightly bigger than normal; the thyroid is, of course, essential for normal postnatal growth.

Placental factors

True placental insufficiency is unlikely to affect the fetus before the 7th month of pregnancy because before that time the functional capacity of the placenta as an exchange organ far exceeds fetal needs. Towards term, however, fetal needs may outstrip the capacity of the placenta, particularly when the placenta begins to undergo degenerative changes associated with fibrin deposition. Most pathological changes in placental function are thought to be secondary to an extraplacental cause.

Maternal factors

These have profound effects on fetal growth:

Parity
Primiparous mothers have smaller babies than multiparous mothers i.e. first babies tend to be smaller than subsequent babies.

Multiple pregnancy
Singletons tend to be larger than twins or triplets. Human fetuses in multiple pregnancies tend to show growth retardation when total fetal weight reaches 3.2 kg, which occurs at the 26th week for quadruplets and the 30th week for twins.

Maternal size
The effect of maternal size on fetal size was demonstrated in Walton and Hammond's classical experiment involving reciprocal crossing between mares and stallions of Shetland ponies and Shire horses; the unequivocal conclusion was that horse fetuses, presumably sharing a similar genetic endowment, grow much faster in the uteri of large mares. In humans birth weight correlates positively with maternal size, though the responsible factors, which may include fetal genotype, maternal nutrition and socio-economic effects, are hard to disentangle.

Maternal age
Teenagers typically have small babies.

Maternal nutrition
Maternal nutrition must obviously, *in extremis*, be a limiting factor on fetal growth, for the fetus must receive a minimum supply of carbohydrate, fat and protein. It is less easy to define the circumstances in which this supply becomes a limiting factor. Effects of maternal nutrition on fetal growth in the sheep are relatively small for the first 3 months of their 5-month pregnancy but ewes fed poorly during the last 2 months of pregnancy give birth to small lambs.

'Good' human data are hard to find, and information derived from starved mothers in Leningrad and Holland during World War II is still quoted. In Leningrad, where conditions were exacerbated by hard work and bitter cold, mean birth weights were reduced by about 550 g but in Holland the reduction was only of the order of 200 g. A high calorie intake during pregnancy in previously malnourished mothers raises mean birth weight; women who are underweight at the start of pregnancy, and continue to restrict their calorie intake, are more likely to have SFD babies.

Maternal socio-economic factors
These are an ill-defined conglomerate which have been alleged to affect birth weight. They include nutrition, housing, health care, sanitation and psychological well-being. Recent studies indicate that variations in birth weight attributed to socio-economic factors are caused by correlated factors rather than by socio-economic status *per se*. A mother's past experience, including her prenatal growth, can influence her ability to provide for her own fetus in utero; thus rats whose diet has been restricted for several generations need more than one generation of adequate nourishment in order for neonates to attain normal size.

Cigarette smoking
Smoking is correlated with socio-economic status in many societies, and adversely affects birth weight, there being a linear dose-response relationship up to a certain level beyond which heavier smoking has little effect. Appetite reduction and uterine vasoconstriction have been said to account for the association between smoking and impaired fetal growth, but it is now believed that the most crucial factor is the high concentration of carboxyhaemoglobin found in the maternal and fetal blood of smoking mothers. The deficit in birth weight may be as high as 300 g, but the mean duration of pregnancy is at most only a day or two shorter than that seen in non-smoking women.

Hypertension and placental blood supply
Maternal hypertension is commonly associated with a reduction in maternal placental blood flow and consequent fetal growth retardation. On the other hand the proportion of larger-than-normal neonates born to women who are hypertensive is also increased. Perhaps certain hypertensive women show an unusually large placental blood flow. Maternal heart disease is also associated with low-birth-weight infants. Experiments in rats demonstrate the

importance of placental blood flow in determining fetal size. Partial occlusion of the arterial supply to one uterine horn causes marked growth retardation in those fetuses which are attached to ischaemic placentae.

Alcohol and drugs
Consumption of alcohol or use of various drugs can cause fetal growth retardation. The head of a baby born to a mother who drinks heavily is typically abnormally small, with deformities which include a flattened facial profile, cleft palate, hare lip and short-sightedness (*fetal alcohol syndrome*).

The circulation

General considerations

1. The placenta, not the lung, is the fetal organ of gaseous exchange. The lungs are solid organs which secrete fluid into the respiratory passages, and extract oxygen from the blood to provide for the metabolic needs of the developing lung tissue. The pulmonary circulation has a high resistance; pulmonary arterioles dilate in response to a rise in P_{O_2} and constrict in response to a rise in P_{CO_2} and/or a fall in pH.

2. Both sides of the heart work in parallel, and total cardiac output is high. Some blood from the inferior vena cava (IVC) passes via the *foramen ovale* to the ascending aorta and the aortic arch; blood from the superior vena cava (SVC), which is less well oxygenated, passes to the descending aorta via the *ductus arteriosus*. This pattern of circulation favours oxygen delivery to the heart and brain at the expense of lower parts of the body.

3. The placenta, not the gut, is the organ of nutrient uptake.

4. Six fetal vascular channels are found which normally obliterate after birth: these are the umbilical vein, two umbilical arteries, the *ductus venosus*, the foramen ovale and the ductus arteriosus.

5. The development of cardiovascular regulatory mechanisms is influenced by the fact that the intrauterine environment is liquid, which reduces sensory input, lessens the need for regulatory mechanisms associated, for example, with temperature or postural changes, and provides an environment favourable for lung development.

The fetal circulation (Fig. 7.3)

Oxygenated blood returning from the placenta in the umbilical vein enters the IVC via the liver and the hepatic veins; about half of it takes a low-resistance bypass through the liver (the *ductus venosus*). The blood passes via the IVC to the right atrium where it is divided into two streams by the free edge of the interatrial septum (the *crista dividens*) which projects from the edge of the foramen ovale. In the lamb fetus it has been shown that only about one-third of the blood in the IVC enters the left atrium directly via the foramen ovale, thus taking the 'via sinistra' (i.e. left route) which bypasses the lungs. In the left atrium the blood is joined by the pulmonary venous return (which is comparatively small), and the 3 per cent of superior vena caval blood which

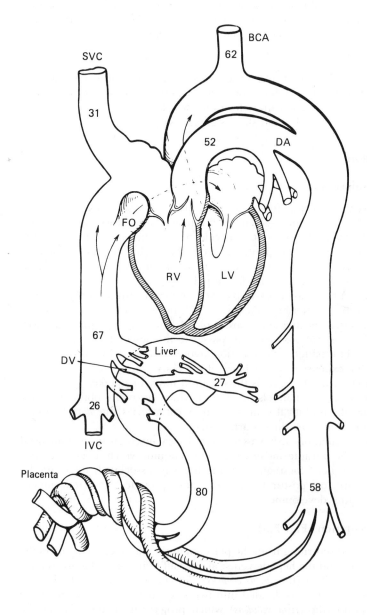

Fig. 7.3 Diagram of the circulation in the fetal lamb. The numerals indicate mean oxygen saturation of the blood sampled from different vessels of six lambs. RV, right ventricle; LV, left ventricle; SVC, superior vena cava; IVC, inferior vena cava; BCA, brachiocephalic artery; FO, foramen ovale; DA, ductus arteriosus; DV, ductus venosus. (From Born, G.V.R., Dawes, G.S., Mott, J.C. and Widdicombe, J.G. (1954). *Cold Spring Harbor Symposia on Quantitative Biology* **19**, 102–108.)

crosses the foramen; both are relatively poorly oxygenated. The areas which receive the blood from the left ventricle are, predominantly, the left myocardium, head, and upper body.

Blood contributing to right heart output, the 'via dextra' (i.e. right route) is made up of two-thirds of the blood from the IVC, together with the bulk of the poorly-oxygenated blood from the SVC. Pulmonary vascular resistance is high, and the fetal lungs receive less than 10 per cent of the total fetal cardiac output (being the combined output of both ventricles). The high resistance results in part from the low fetal pulmonary oxygen tension — 20–25 mmHg, compared with 80–100 mmHg in the adult. Pulmonary arterioles are unusual in that they constrict when oxygen tension is low so that pulmonary resistance is increased by fetal hypoxia. Pulmonary arterial pressure is higher in the fetus than systemic arterial pressure. The consequence is that the bulk of the output of the right heart enters the widely open ductus arteriosus to pass into the descending aorta where it joins what remains of the blood from the left heart which has not passed to the head and upper body. About half of the combined left and right heart output in the human passes to the placenta.

The walls of the right and left ventricles of the fetal heart are about equally thick until about half-way through pregnancy, but in the second half of gestation the right ventricular myocardium becomes relatively thicker; outflow from this ventricle passes mainly to the lower half of the body, and through the very long umbilical arteries to the placenta. The fetal heart rate is about 65/min in the 15 mm embryo, reaching a peak rate of 175/min at the ninth week. From mid-term onwards the normal range is between 135 and 155/min.

The fetal heart is susceptible to autonomic control quite early in gestation, and baroreceptor reflexes are well developed at birth. Maternal hypoxia, occlusion of the umbilical cord, and compression of the fetal head all cause reflex bradycardia which could serve to reduce cardiac work and expenditure of cardiac carbohydrate reserves. Persistent bradycardia before delivery is a sign of fetal hypoxia which can have serious consequences for the development of the central nervous system.

Changes in the fetal circulation at the time of birth (Fig. 7.4)

The characteristics of the neonatal circulation are as follows:

Pulmonary vascular resistance

The low resistance placental circulation is lost, but a low resistance pulmonary circulation is gained. Pulmonary arterial pressures do not, however, fall immediately, and equal or exceed those in the systemic aorta in many subjects during the first hour post-partum. A decline in pulmonary arterial pressure occurs during the first 2 to 3 days of life, the rate of decline being related to the rate of closure of the ductus arteriosus. Early clamping of the umbilical cord is associated with lower pulmonary arterial pressure after birth. In infants born at high altitude, where the Po_2 will be lower, pulmonary vascular resistance is higher and remains higher for longer.

Closure of the ductus arteriosus
At term the external diameter of the ductus is about 6 mm, and its length 1.25 cm. It closes in two stages; the first is a rapid post-partum constriction apparently caused by the direct effect of high Po_2 on smooth muscle of the ductus.

Prostaglandins and/or prostacyclins are probably involved in the closure of the ductus — perhaps as mediators of the effect of oxygen. Later anatomical obliteration may take weeks or months and during this period the constricted duct may re-open if pulmonary vascular resistance increases owing to hypoxia or hypercapnia.

Placental transfusion
At the moment of birth the placenta contains about 125 ml of blood, which is about a third of the fetal blood volume. Placental separation typically occurs

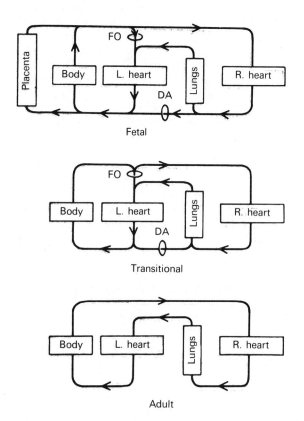

Fetal

Transitional

Adult

Fig. 7.4 Diagrams showing transition from parallel to series pattern of blood flow through heart as the fetal circulation passes via a transitional stage to the adult arrangement. Abbreviations as in Fig. 7.3. (From Born, G.V.R., Dawes, G.S., Mott, J.C. and Widdicombe, J.G. (1954). *Cold Spring Harbor Symposia on Quantitative Biology* **19**, 102–108.)

2–4 minutes later, and during this period, a substantial volume of blood passes from placenta to fetus — enough to provide for the infant's oxygen needs at this crucial time; oxygen, carbon dioxide and pH levels in the blood of the neonate are unchanged prior to the first breath unless there is placental separation, or the umbilical cord is prematurely clamped. The rate at which blood passes from the placenta to the newborn infant depends upon several factors including gravity and uterine contraction. Premature clamping will result in a residue of blood remaining in the placenta, and this may impede placental separation by preventing the reduction in size of the subplacental area of uterine wall which is an important determinant of complete placental separation. On the other hand, delayed cord clamping may impose a strain on the neonatal cardiovascular system.

The foramen ovale
The transformation of the heart from working as two pumps in parallel to working as two pumps in series depends on the closure of the foramen ovale. This has a diameter of 8 mm at term and a loose valve on the left atrial side permits flow only from the IVC into the left atrium. With the first breath, pulmonary vascular resistance decreases. This results in an increase in pulmonary blood flow, and pulmonary venous flow to the left atrium increases causing a rise in left atrial pressure. Coupled with this is a fall in right atrial pressure resulting from a fall in IVC pressure caused by the reduction in umbilical venous flow. The reversal of pressure difference between the atria causes rapid functional closure of the foramen ovale, though anatomical closure takes a minimum of 3 months, and may take a year or more; indeed one can pass a probe through the foramen ovale in more than 10 per cent of adults.

Size of the ventricles
The newborn has a relatively high pulmonary vascular pressure and resistance, but this declines and pulmonary blood flow increases; systemic pressure and resistance, on the other hand, rise. The cardiac output of the newborn is two to three times higher than that of the adult if expressed in terms of body weight. At birth, the right ventricular wall is thicker than the left, but this situation gradually reverses, reflecting the altered workload on the two ventricles in postnatal life. Adult ventricular weight relationships are attained within the first 10 months.

Cardiovascular control mechanisms
Baroreceptor and chemoreceptor cardiovascular reflexes are active in the neonate. The neonate is susceptible to significant departures from normal blood volume which, if they arise, can cause haemodynamic effects which may disrupt the normal closure of the two left-right shunts (ductus arteriosus and foramen ovale). Normally the rates of closure of the various fetal vessels are appropriate to permit smooth alterations in the volume and direction of flow in the shunts.

The lungs

The fetal lung

Primitive air sacs begin to develop from the bronchial tree of the fetus from about the 20th week and lung mesenchyme is invaded by blood vessels by about the 28th week. Development and proliferation of alveoli continues for many months after birth. Fetal lungs are fluid-filled; this fluid contributes to amniotic fluid, but differs from it in having a low pH and CO_2 content.

Crucial to the filling of alveoli with air at birth is the production during fetal life of agents (*surfactants*) which reduce the surface tension of lung fluid and thus reduce the pressure of air required to expand the lungs. Lining cells of the alveoli develop osmiophilic inclusion bodies composed of phospholipids — in particular dipalmitoylphosphatidylcholine (dipalmitoyl-lecithin or DPL) and phosphatidylglycerol. Enzymes needed to synthesize these surfactant substances are found in the fetal lung between the 18th and 20th week, but increase markedly in quantity in the last month or two of gestation. Synthesis depends on rising fetal corticosteroid levels towards the end of pregnancy, and can be accelerated in the fetal sheep by administration of corticosteroids to the mother. If surfactant is produced in insufficient quantity (and it seems likely that *both* DPL and phosphatidylglycerol are needed for optimal effect) normal expansion of the newborn lung is impossible, causing the *idiopathic respiratory distress syndrome (IRDS)* also known as *hyaline membrane disease (HMD)*, because of the clear exudate found in affected alveoli examined under the microscope (Steele: *Gynaecology, Obstetrics and the Neonate*, Chapter 5). The fetal lung cannot, in the event of premature delivery, achieve gaseous exchange adequate to support life until about the 26th week, and even then is ill-prepared for proper function. Prior to the 26th week alveoli are inadequately developed and the air-capillary barrier is too thick to permit adequate gas exchange.

Fetal respiratory movements are detectable in the human by the 11th week. They have been shown to occur in the fetal lamb when the electroencephalographic activity is typical of that found in 'REM' sleep. Initially they are irregular, but their regularity increases throughout gestation until just prior to labour. In the lamb they cause just 1 ml of to-and-fro movement in the trachea — insufficient to clear the tracheal dead space. Respiratory movements increase if the fetal P_{CO_2} rises, but decrease if the fetus becomes either hypoxic (which may happen if the mother smokes cigarettes) or hypoglycaemic. Fetal carotid chemoreceptors seem to be much less sensitive than those in the adult, for no chemoreceptor activity can be recorded in the sheep fetal carotid sinus nerve over a range of P_{O_2} from 10–200 mmHg. Aortic chemoreceptors are active in the fetal sheep at term, but the reflex consequences of their stimulation are circulatory rather than respiratory; hypoxia causes peripheral vasoconstriction and raises blood pressure — so diverting blood to the brain — the organ most threatened by hypoxia.

Initiation of breathing

The first breath must overcome surface tension, the viscosity of fluid in the airway, and tissue resistance (Steele: *Gynaecology, Obstetrics and the Neonate*,

Chapter 4): Lung fluid is expressed during normal vaginal delivery by the high pressure exerted on the thorax. The removal of the remaining fluid via the pulmonary capillaries (and to a lesser extent by the lymphatics) is accelerated by adrenaline which is released by the fetus in response to the stress of parturition; fluid removal is largely complete by 1 hour postpartum.

Aeration of the lungs is achieved in part by elastic recoil following the release of the compression of the thorax during birth. Contraction of the diaphragm results in inspiration of 30–70 ml of air most of which remains in the lung to form part of the residual volume, which increases with subsequent breaths. Inspiratory pressure initially must be large, but a steadily decreasing effort is required for subsequent breaths (Fig 7.5). With the onset of air-breathing, pulmonary vascular resistance falls owing to the rise in Po_2 and physical expansion of the lungs.

What mechanisms bring about the pronounced inspiratory effort which is so vital to the survival of the newborn baby?

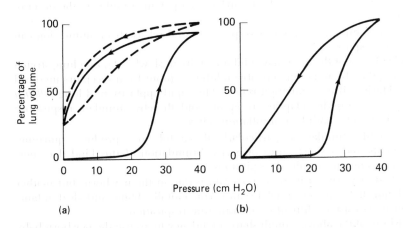

Fig. 7.5 Loops constructed by plotting lung volume against the pressure required to inflate and deflate (a) mature and (b) immature fetal lungs in the lamb. The continuous line in (a) represents the first breath and the dotted line represents subsequent breaths. The initial inflation of the mature fetal lungs requires a large pressure because they are collapsed and fluid-filled at the start, but during deflation the lungs remain much more inflated and subsequent inflations require very little pressure. In the immature fetus a similar initial inflating pressure is required, but on deflation the lungs collapse completely and each subsequent inflation requires the same high pressure as the first; a comparable situation arises in infants with respiratory distress syndrome. (From Reynolds, E.O.R. and Strang, B. (1966). *British Medical Bulletin* **22**, 79–83.)

Chemoreceptor activation

A degree of asphyxiation is normal during birth, resulting in a fall in arterial Po_2 and a rise in Pco_2. The resulting acidosis is partly respiratory and partly metabolic, the latter arising from the accumulation of the products of anaerobic glycolysis. In the fetal lamb, sympathetic activation follows asphyxia; this constricts arterioles, including those to the carotid body. The resulting decrease in carotid body blood flow may increase chemoreceptor sensitivity to both low P_{O_2} and high P_{CO_2}. Breathing can, however, be initiated in newborn lambs after section of the carotid sinus nerves; peripheral chemoreceptors are therefore not essential for the initiation of breathing. Central chemoreceptors respond to a fall of brain extracellullar fluid pH such as would be caused by a rise in arterial P_{CO_2}, and they probably contribute to the respiratory drive resulting from neonatal asphyixa. The newborn is, however, sensitive to arterial P_{O_2}, and depression of respiration may occur, sometimes even apnoea, if a newborn baby is given 100 per cent oxygen to breathe. The initial response of the newborn to hypoxia is an initial period of apnoea, followed by about 2 minutes of gasping, after which a period of 'terminal' apnoea precedes death. The duration of the initial apnoeic response is increased by opiates.

Non-chemical stimuli

(a) Cooling of the face or body surface is a potent stimulus to the onset of breathing.

(b) Facial immersion inhibits respiration, and release from immersion can stimulate respiration.

(c) Deflation of the lung may inhibit activity in slowly adapting lung stretch receptors thereby removing possible inhibitory input from receptors involved in the Hering–Breuer inflation reflex. The rapid application of lung *inflation* may activate rapidly-adapting receptors and thereby stimulate respiratory effort via Head's paradoxical inflation reflex.

(d) Tactile stimulation, particularly if painful, may produce squirming movements and a short series of gasps. Stimulation of this kind does not, however, generate sustained respiration.

(e) Auditory stimuli increase respiratory rate in the newborn, but neither sound nor light are essential because congenitally blind and deaf infants exhibit no consistent difficulties in initiating respiration.

(f) Many of the above stimuli share a tendency to arouse the newborn baby from the behaviourally dull, unresponsive, 'obtunded' state which commonly persists until umbilical blood flow is occluded. At this point, and the process can be observed very clearly in the lamb, the newborn writhes, shakes, muscle tone increases and sympathetico-adrenal activation occurs. Onset of respiration may be just one component of this generalized postpartum arousal.

Conclusion

Many factors, then, contribute to the onset of the first breath. They operate on a newborn organism in which the neuromuscular relationships between swallowing and breathing are established, pulmonary stretch receptors are functional, medullary respiratory rhythmicity is established, and irritants and foreign bodies in the pharynx and trachea can be detected. Thus the passage of the fetus 'through the valley of the shadow of birth' is assured.

Bilirubin metabolism

Bilirubin is formed in fetus, neonate and adult as a result of haemoglobin catabolism in cells of liver, spleen and kidney. In these cells microsomal haem oxygenase causes the loss by haemoglobin of its globulin and ferric iron, yielding *biliverdin* which then becomes bilirubin (Fig. 7.6). Bilirubin, a lipid-soluble derivative of protoporphyrin IX, is present in plasma either free, or bound to plasma proteins and, to a lesser exent, to red blood cells. If all binding sites are occupied more bilirubin circulates in the free state and, being lipid-soluble, can migrate across the blood-brain barrier to cause *kernicterus* or *bilirubin encephalopathy* which can result in severe and lasting damage to the developing central nervous system.

Bilirubin in the fetus is normally present in lower concentrations, and moves freely across the placenta into the maternal circulation (Fig 7.6). This simple means for disposing of bilirubin is unavailable to the newborn, causing the danger of a rapid rise in free plasma bilirubin concentration. This danger is met by the gradual development, within the neonatal liver, of the

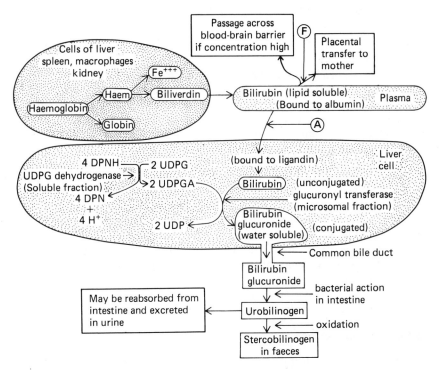

Fig. 7.6 Diagram showing the formation of bilirubin by haemoglobin catabolism. In the fetus it is excreted by diffusion across the placenta to the maternal circulation (the route marked 'F'). Bilirubin glucuronide passes slowly across the placenta and its synthesis is therefore suppressed in the fetus, but after birth the placenta ceases to be available and bilirubin must then be excreted via conjugation in the liver (the route marked 'A') which is the adult excretory mechanism.

wherewithal to bind bilirubin within liver cells (the protein *ligandin*), to synthesize uridinediphosphate-glucuronic acid (UDPGA) for UDP glucose and diphosphonucleoside (DPN)(UPDG dehydrogenase), and to achieve the conjugation of bilirubin to glucuronide (glucuronyl transferase). Conjugated bilirubin is excreted by the liver via the common bile duct. The system for conjugating bilirubin is normally activated only after birth because, once conjugated, bilirubin cannot cross the placenta. The suppression of bilirubin conjugation in the fetus may be associated with the presence in maternal plasma of progestational steroids — in particular pregnanediol. Pregnanediol can inhibit conjugation of bilirubin by liver slices in vitro, and may be present in breast milk for a week or two postpartum when it may contribute to a mild self-limiting hyperbilirubinaemia in the breast-fed infant.

Physiological hyperbilirubinaemia

A mild *physiological* hyperbilirubinaemia (called *jaundice*, because of the resulting yellow colouration of skin and mucous membranes) is quite common in newborn infants (Steele: *Gynaecology, Obstetrics and the Neonate*, Chapter 5) and the following factors may contribute to its occurrence:

1. The shorter life-span of red cells in the newborn (60–70 days) compared with the adult (100–120 days). The life-span in the premature infant may be as low as 30–40 days.

2. If the newborn infant has an unusually large blood volume the rate of red cell breakdown may be accelerated. This can arise if the umbilical cord is clamped later rather than sooner: 5 per cent of babies in which the cord is clamped early show jaundice, whereas it is seen in 30 per cent of babies in which the cord is clamped late. If the infant is bruised during parturition, this too may result in haemoglobin breakdown at a greater rate than normal.

3. Dehydration and/or insufficient caloric intake (with or without hypoglycaemia) tend to be associated with a low rate of bilirubin conjugation. Such conditions are physiological in the breast-fed baby whose intake of water and calories is low for the first 2 or 3 days after birth.

4. Bilirubin conjugation may be depressed by physiological inhibitors, such as the steroid hormones mentioned above.

5. In the early weeks after birth, the infant has low levels of ligandin in liver cells and a slightly deficient execretory mechanism for the disposal of conjugated bilirubin.

6. The above factors are exacerbated in the premature baby in whom bilirubin conjugation develops particularly slowly.

Other liver functions

Enzymes concerned in bilirubin metabolism are not the only liver enzymes which must become active at or about the end of gestation. Enzymes concerned with amino acid biosynthesis and nitrogen excretion are needed for postnatal life (e.g. tyrosine alphaketoglutarate transaminase). In many cases, their synthesis and activity is controlled by hormones such as glucagon (which itself increases postnatally in response to hypoglycaemia) and glucocorticoids.

Tyrosine oxidizing enzymes are deficient in the liver of premature babies, which may be prone to hypertyrosinaemia particularly on a diet high in protein and low in vitamin C; minimal brain damage may possibly result. Cystathionase activity is absent in the fetus, suggesting that the fetus depends entirely on the mother for its supply of cystine and cysteine. For premature infants these amino acids are probably essential until some time after birth. Human milk is a good source of cystine, whereas cow's milk is not; furthermore cow's milk can cause the accumulation of methionine in premature infants.

Kidney function

Fetal kidney function

The definitive excretory organ of the human derives from the metanephros, which, in ontogeny as in phylogeny, follows the earlier pronephros and mesonephros. The total adult complement of nephrons is achieved by about the 36th week of fetal life, though many will at that stage be immature. Although renal blood flow in the sheep fetus is relatively low (only 2 per cent of cardiac output compared with about 25 per cent in the adult), there is an appreciable output of urine; the glomerular filtration rate is also low, but this is offset by a lower renal tubular reabsorption of sodium than in the adult. Amniotic fluid is largely derived from fetal urine, which no doubt accounts for its increasing concentrations of creatinine and urea. Amniotic fluid is hypotonic compared with maternal plasma by about 27 mosmols/kg, and this must be due, at least in part, to a regular outpouring of fetal urine which plays an important part in the maintenance of amniotic fluid volume. Renal agenesis (*Potter's syndrome*) results in a lack of amniotic fluid, but need not cause fetal death because the fetus is constantly being haemodialysed by the placenta. The fetal kidney may play some part in the regulation of fetal growth, blood pressure and potassium homoeostasis.

Postnatal transition in kidney function

The fetal kidney, then, produces large quantities of urine regardless of the cost in loss of salt and water; ample replacements are available from the mother via the placenta, as well as by recycling of the sodium and water excreted into the amniotic fluid and swallowed by the fetus. At birth the kidney must suddenly reduce the loss of fluid and electrolyte to balance the much reduced supply. The problem has been graphically described as 'emergence from the primeval swamp to the extrauterine desert'.

In the first few hours of extrauterine life, there is a high rate of urine flow and a relatively low rate of sodium reabsorption. In the next few hours, urine flow rate falls rapidly to rise again at the end of the first week. Glomerular filtration rate in the kidney of the new born is low, about a third to a quarter of what would be expected in relation to body size. It rises to 'normal' by the second year of life, perhaps because of glomerular maturation and a rising arterial blood pressure.

Tubular function in the neonatal kidney is deficient. The newborn baby can neither excrete an excessive load of sodium (so may become oedematous when fed a saline solution), nor retain sodium (and is thus in danger of hyponatraemia); the latter danger is increased in premature babies whose kidneys leak sodium at three times the rate of those of full-term infants (Steele: *Gynaecology, Obstetrics and the Neonate*, Chapter 5). The concentrating power of neonatal kidneys is deficient and they can achieve a maximum urine concentration of only 700–800 mosmol/kg compared with the 1200–1400 mosmol/kg in the older child and adult. The main reason for this poor performance is the low level of production and excretion of urea by the growing baby who, if placed on a diet very high in protein, or given urea by mouth, can produce a urine almost as concentrated as that of the adult. The role of urea in urine concentration depends upon its being re-cycled by the various ducts and blood vessels found in the renal medulla. The infant can produce as dilute a urine as the adult (about 50 mosmols/kg), but the rate of excretion of a water load is lower.

The low level of tubular reabsorption of sodium may contribute to an abnormally large loss of sodium bicarbonate in newborn babies which, even though they may be acidaemic, tend to excrete a urine of inappropriately high pH during the first week or two after birth. Aldosterone is needed by newborn babies; if it is deficient (as in 21-hydroxylase deficiency), untreated babies may die at the age of a week from hyponatraemia, dehydration and hyperkalaemia.

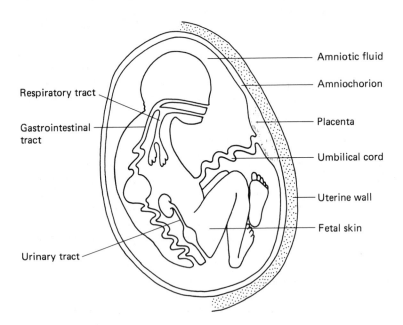

Fig. 7.7 Pathways involved in the formation of amniotic fluid. The placenta, umbilical cord and amniochorion exchange materials continuously. Fetal skin exchanges materials up to the time of keratinization, after which the kidneys are the major source of fluid.

The fetal fluids

The fetus is surrounded by membrane-bound fluid-filled cavities. In many species there are two cavities — *allantoic* and *amniotic* — but in the human only the amniotic cavity need be considered.

Formation and reabsorption of amniotic fluid ('liquor amnii')(Fig. 7.7)

The amniotic cavity is not a stagnant pool used for the excretion of urine; there is a complete exchange of amniotic fluid water about every 3 hours. For about the first 20 weeks of gestation, the skin of the fetus is not keratinized and amniotic fluid can exchange freely with, and is effectively an extension of, the fetal extracellular fluid. During this time amniotic fluid has an osmolarity of about 300 mosmols/litre.

With the keratinization of the fetal skin, what remaining sites may add or remove components of the amniotic fluid? Hypotonic urine is excreted into the amniotic cavity (at rates of up to 500 ml/day in the fetal sheep), and the fetus swallows amniotic fluid at about the same rate. The fetal stomach can absorb sodium against a concentration gradient and is likely to be an

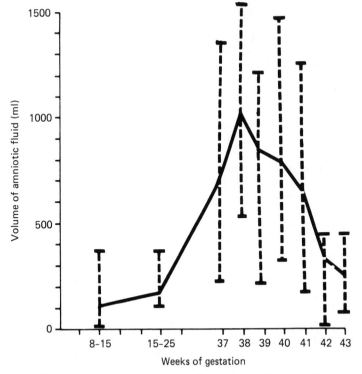

Fig. 7.8 Volume (averages and ranges) of amniotic fluid from the 16th to the 43rd week of pregnancy demonstrating the large variations between individuals. Volume peaks several weeks before term, and falls rapidly as term approaches. (From Kerpel-Fronius, E. (1978). In: *Perinatal Physiology*. Ed. by U. Stave. Plenum, New York.)

important site of amniotic fluid reabsorption. The fetal gut does not appear to act as a source of amniotic fluid, but particularly towards term, the fetal lungs may produce fluid at a significant rate; this no doubt explains the presence of pulmonary surfactant in amniotic fluid in late pregnancy. The pattern of change of amniotic fluid volume during pregnancy is shown in Fig. 7.8.

The amniotic cavity is limited externally by the *amniochorion*, and fluid may move across this membrane, being driven by both osmotic and hydrostatic forces. Normally flow is believed to be outwards from the amniotic cavity and the rate of flow may be accelerated by making the mother hypertonic. Part of the outer border of the amniotic cavity forms the fetal surface of the placenta; this interface is a site for exchange of water, sodium, chloride, urea and creatinine between amniotic fluid and fetal blood.

To summarize, the principal source of amniotic fluid is the fetal kidneys; if they fail to develop (*Potter's syndrome*) *oligohydramnios* (insufficient amniotic fluid) will be the result. Since amniotic fluid is removed through the fetal gut, *hydramnios* (or *polyhydramnios*), i.e. excessive accumulation of amniotic fluid, results when swallowing fails owing to oesophageal atresia or anencephaly (Steele: *Gynaecology, Obstetrics and the Neonate*, Chapter 10).

Composition of amniotic fluid (Table 7.1)

Collection of amniotic fluid by amniocentesis is common obstetric practice, and the detection and/or estimation of constituents of amniotic fluid is valuable in determining fetal well-being (Steele: *Gynaecology, Obstetrics and the Neonate*, Chapter 1). Early in pregnancy, amniotic fluid resembles fetal extracellular fluid. As pregnancy advances, osmolarity declines, sodium concentration falls, and concentration of non-protein nitrogenous compounds, notably urea and creatinine, rises. The total protein concentration is about one-tenth that of serum, and fibrinogen is absent. Albumin and globulin concentration are roughly the same as those found in serum. Glucose concentration tends to be lower than that in maternal serum. Hormones are detectable: oestrogens increase sharply during the last trimester, and hCG, pregnanediol, progesterone, 17-ketosteroids, hPL and prolactin are also found. About 30 different enzymes can be detected, and their analysis may assist in the early diagnosis of inborn errors of metabolism. There are four components of amniotic fluid the analysis of which has assumed particular clinical importance:

1. α-*fetoprotein* is a glycoprotein (mol. wt approx 70 000) which is present in maximal concentration in the serum of the 16 week fetus; it persists in fetal serum up to term, but declines rapidly postpartum. Its concentration in amniotic fluid in the second half of pregnancy is normally very low, but is raised both in amniotic fluid and in maternal serum if the fetal skin is broken, as would be the case in anencephaly or spina bifida.

2. About half the *lipids* in amniotic fluid are fatty acids, but towards term the phospholipid DPL (a pulmonary surfactant) appears in increasing quantities.

3. Fetal, but not maternal, *cells* may be found in amniotic fluid and

Table 7.1 Compositions of amniotic fluid in early and late pregnancy and the full-term maternal and fetal serum. (From Biggers, J.D. (1980). In: *Medical Physiology*, vol. 2, 14th edn. Ed. by V.B. Mountcastle. C.V. Mosby, St Louis; modified from Seeds, A.E. (1972). In: *The Water Metabolism of the Fetus*, Ed. by A.C. Barnes and A.E. Seeds, Charles Thomas, Springfield, Illinois)

Fluid	Total osmotic pressure (mosmols)	Na (mM)	Cl (mM)	K (mM)	NPN (mg/ 100 ml)	Urea (mg/ 100 ml)	Uric acid (mg/ 100 ml)	Creatinine (mg/ 100 ml)	Total protein (mg/ 100ml)	Water content (%)
Amniotic fluid, first and second trimester	283	134	110	4.2	24	25	3.2	1.23	0.28	98.7
Amniotic fluid, third trimester	262	126	105	4.0	27	34	5.6	2.17	0.26	98.8
Maternal serum, full-term	289	137	105	3.6	22	21	—	1.55	6.5	91.6
Fetal serum, full-term	290	140	106	4.5	23	25	3.6	1.02	5.5	—

chromosomal analysis may reveal abnormalities such as Down's syndrome. Examination of the cells may also enable the sex of an unborn child to be determined, which may be valuable in families with a history of sex-linked hereditary disorders.

4. *Bilirubin* levels rise in amniotic fluid in cases of haemolytic disease of the newborn.

Fetal and neonatal endocrinology

Few hormones other than unconjugated steroids cross the placenta. In the fetus, most endocrine glands are developed within the first 6 weeks of conception and become functional between the sixth and tenth week; most hormones are detectable in the fetal circulation by the 12th week.

Hypothalamic-pituitary function

The anterior pituitary gland develops from *Rathke's pouch* which is formed from ectoderm in the roof of the buccal cavity. By the 11th week acidophilic and basophilic cells are distinguishable. The hypothalamic-pituitary portal vascular system is developed by the 15th week, and concurrently hypothalamic nuclei are developed containing neurotransmitters such as dopamine, noradrenaline and serotonin and hormones such as thyrotrophin-releasing hormone (TRH) and gonadotrophin-releasing hormone (GnRH). Fetal anterior pituitary endocrine function passes through three stages during gestation: initially hypothalamic and pituitary hormones are secreted independently, after which pituitary hormone secretion is stimulated by uninhibited secretion of hypothalamic hormones. Neural inhibition of hypothalamic-pituitary activity develops during the last trimester.

Human growth hormone (hGH; somatotrophin)
Growth hormone is necessary for normal growth in infants, children and adolescents, but its biological role in the fetus is not clear. Maternal hGH appears not to cross the placenta and does not influence the fetus. The concentration of hGH in the fetal plasma rises until about the fifth month of gestation, and then declines throughout the rest of gestation. Measurements of fetal weight and length in anencephalic fetuses indicate that hGH is not needed for fetal growth, but more careful analysis of individual organ weights and cell numbers indicate that anterior pituitary hormones, including hGH, may play some part in the control of fetal growth. Decapitation of the fetal rabbit does not, according to Jost, impair fetal growth; growth is however impaired in decapitated rat and mouse fetuses, and in hypophysectomized sheep fetuses.

Prolactin
Small amounts of maternal prolactin may enter the fetal circulation, and prolactin is found in amniotic fluid in concentrations 100 times greater than those in either mother or fetus; this amniotic prolactin is probably derived mainly from the fetus. After the 30th week fetal plasma levels rise sharply until

term. After a very brief postpartum rise, plasma concentrations in the neonate decline to steady values by the sixth week postpartum. There is no shortage of suggestions, but scant evidence, for biological roles of prolactin in the fetus.

The gonadotrophins

Serum luteinizing hormone (LH) in the fetus rises to high levels (comparable with those in the castrate) prior to the 20th week, being higher in the female fetus than in the male (see Fig. 1.4). Levels then fall and LH is undetectable in umbilical cord blood at term. In the first weeks postpartum LH levels are high, rising to a maximun at one month, and then falling to low prepubertal levels during the first year of life. Lutinizing hormone levels are greater in male than in female infants.

Follicle-stimulating hormone (FSH) may rise to high levels in the serum of female fetuses between the 12th and the 20th week, but is low and often undetectable in male fetuses during this period. After the 20th week FSH levels fall and are very low in the neonate. Follicle-stimulating hormone levels rise in neonates until about the third month of life and fall to prepubertal levels by 2 years of age.

Though it is not a fetal pituitary hormone, human chorionic gonadotrophin (hCG) should be mentioned; though present between the 12th and 20th weeks in the fetal circulation in concentrations only one-thirtieth of those in the mother, it is believed to have an important role in the male fetus in stimulating interstitial (Leydig) cells of the testis to produce the androgens which are crucial in early sexual differentiation.

Fetal gonads (Fig. 1.4)

Testes

Serum testosterone levels are highest during the period between the 11th and 17th week; during that time they often reach the same values as those found in the adult male. After the 17th week testosterone levels decline. In female fetuses testosterone levels are much lower and do not change in mid-gestation. At birth, levels of free testosterone, i.e. not bound to the sex-hormone binding globulin, are three times as great as those found in adults; the biological activity of all this androgen is probably impeded both by the capacity of the placenta to aromatize testosterone to oestrogens, and by the 'protective' effect of high levels of fetal oestradiol at that time. Testicular androgen production occurs in fetuses at term, and within hours of birth plasma testosterone concentrations rise rapidly (to about eight times the levels in cord serum) in male neonates. Peak levels are reached in males between one and two months of age, and then decline until, by 7 months, they are in the prepubertal range. The sex-hormone binding globulin is present in fairly low plasma levels at birth, but these rise rapidly; despite the rise, free testosterone levels in male babies between the first and second month of life are 40 times greater than those in female babies, and are in the range found in mid-puberty.

Ovaries

The fetal ovaries play no part in the control of sexual differentiation, for the sexual differentiation of the female fetus is a passive process. Fetal oestradiol levels show no difference between male and female fetuses, suggesting that the fetal ovaries are not the source of the hormone; nonetheless fetal FSH and LH levels are both elevated in the female fetus, and fetal ovarian follicles grow and differentiate, indicating that the hypothalamic-pituitary ovarian axis is not dormant in the female fetus.

The thyroid gland

There is a progressive rise in human fetal plasma thyroxine (T4) concentration from about the 20th week of gestation; at term, fetal T4 concentration may exceed that found in maternal serum. By the 11th week of intrauterine life, the fetal thyroid can concentrate iodine and secrete thyroid hormones; at the same time thyroid stimulating hormone (TSH) is detectable in fetal serum. Additional fetal thyroid stimulation may arise from placental *human chorionic thyrotrophin (hCT)*, a glycoprotein which structurally resembles bovine TSH. Fetal tri-iodothyronine is present in low concentrations; the fetus appears to deiodinate T4 preferentially to *reverse tri-iodothyoronine (rT3)* which, though present in high levels in the fetus, is metabolically inactive. Plasma TSH levels rise sharply after birth.

Adequate fetal thyroxine levels are necessary for normal fetal development, including the production of pulmonary surfactant. The fetus depends in part on the adequate function of its own thyroid gland but placental permeability to thyroxine increases during the second half of pregnancy, so that maternal thyroid hormone potentially becomes available to the fetus near term. Absence of thyroid tissue in the fetus therefore has relatively minor effects — on the basis of clinical examination of the newborn infant; however, if vigorous therapy with thyroid hormones is not instituted, the somatic and psychological features of cretinism soon appear.

The pituitary-adrenal cortex axis

The human fetal adrenal cortex appears during the fourth week of gestation. It is composed of two distinct zones. The inner fetal zone accounts for 85 per cent of the mass of the fetal adrenal cortex and is composed of large eosinophilic cells. The outer zone is composed of undifferentiated, and probably nonfunctional, cells. The outer zone shows enlargement and proliferation after birth; by the fourth postpartum day, the inner zone begins to degenerate. A distinct fetal zone is present only in the human, the chimpanzee and, to some extent, the rhesus monkey, and its significance for fetal development is not clear. Although the growth of the fetal zone during the second half of pregnancy is ACTH-dependent, its development during the first half of pregnancy is independent of ACTH, for adrenals grow normally during this time in anencephalic fetuses. Fetal adrenal growth coincides with increased concentration of prolactin in fetal plasma, and a corticotrophic role for fetal prolactin has been suggested.

Pituitary ACTH and related hormones
Adrenocorticotrophic hormone (ACTH) is a straight-chain 39-amino-acid peptide. It is synthesized as a larger molecule, 'big ACTH', which may be the

precursor for various peptides including ACTH, β-lipotrophin, β-melanocyte-stimulating hormone (β-MSH), and corticotrophin-like intermediate lobe peptide (CLIP). The human fetal pituitary contains relatively large quantities of these small ACTH fragments, but at birth ACTH becomes predominant. These fragments may specifically stimulate the growth of the fetal zone of the adrenal cortex. Fetal plasma ACTH levels are fairly high during the 12th to 19th week and decrease by the 35th to 40th week; they are rather variable, but often very high, in umbilical cord blood samples at term. Levels are higher in the umbilical artery than in the umbilical vein, suggesting that fetal ACTH is secreted endogenously and is not derived from the maternal circulation by transplacental passage. The high levels of ACTH in the term fetus after vaginal delivery probably reflect secretion of the hormone in response to the stress of parturition.

The feto-placental unit
The fetal adrenal cortex and the placenta function during pregnancy as a steroid synthesizing unit (the *feto-placental unit*), the biochemical functions of the one complementing those of the other. The fetal adrenal cortex is deficient in 3 β-hydroxysteroid dehydrogenase (3 β-HSD), and Δ^5 isomerase, while the placenta lacks C_{17-20} lyase (also known as C_{17-20} desmolase), which is present in the fetal adrenal gland.

The synthesis of oestrogens by the feto-placental unit (Fig. 7.9a) begins with the conversion in the fetal adrenal of cholesterol to pregnenolone; the supply of cholesterol presents no problem, for most fetal tissues can synthesize cholesterol from glucose or acetate, and cholesterol may also pass from mother to fetus across the placenta. From pregnenolone the fetal adrenal cortex synthesizes dehydroepiandrosterone (DHEA) and its sulphate (DHEAS), and these substances pass to the placenta to serve as precursors for synthesis of oestrone and oestradiol. Dehydroepiandrosterone sulphate may also pass to the fetal liver where it encounters 16α-hydroxylase which converts it to 16α-hydroxydehydroepiandrosterone sulphate which passes to the placenta to serve as a precursor for oestriol synthesis.

The fetal adrenal is not the sole source of precursors for placental synthesis of oestrogens. The maternal adrenal also synthesizes DHEA which is converted to oestradiol by the placenta, and this will be 16 α-hydroxylated in the maternal liver to oestriol. Maternal urinary oestriol levels are thus an imperfect, albeit a useful, indicator of fetal adrenal function.

There is a second set of synthetic pathways in which the activities of fetal adrenal and placenta are complementary (Fig. 7.9b); in this case it is the placenta which provides the precursor needed for the later stages of the synthetic activity which occur in the fetal adrenal cortex. The placenta produces pregnenolone from cholesterol, and has the 3 β-HSD necessary for the conversion of pregnenolone to progesterone. Much of this progesterone enters the maternal circulation, but some enters the fetal circulation where it serves as an essential precursor for the elaboration of deoxycorticosterone, corticosterone, cortisol and aldosterone by the fetal adrenal cortex. The placenta itself cannot synthesize these steroids because it lacks the necessary 21-, 11 β-, 17α-, and 18-hydroxylase enzymes. Some cortisol may pass from

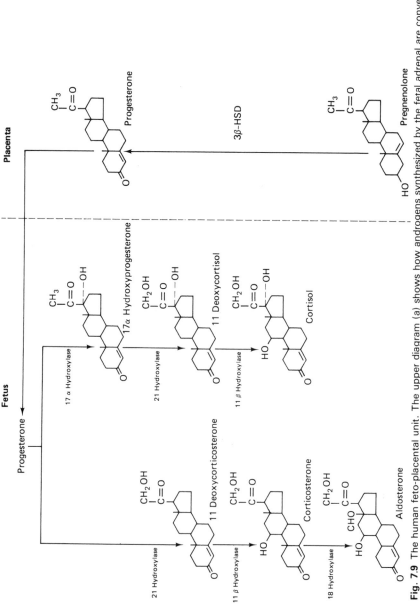

Fig. 7.9 The human feto-placental unit. The upper diagram (a) shows how androgens synthesized by the fetal adrenal are converted to oestrogens which appear in large quantities in the maternal circulation. The lower diagram (b) shows how progesterone synthesized by the placenta is converted to mineralocorticoids and glucocorticoids by the fetal adrenal. (From Silman, R.E., Chard, T. and Boyd, N.R.H. (1977). In: *Scientific Foundations of Obstetrics and Gynaecology*, 2nd edn. Ed. by E.E. Philipp, J. Barnes and M. Newton. Heinemann, London.)

Placenta

Progesterone

3β-HSD

Pregnenolone

Fetus

Progesterone

17 α Hydroxylase

17α Hydroxyprogesterone

21 Hydroxylase

11 Deoxycortisol

11 β Hydroxylase

Cortisol

21 Hydroxylase

11 Deoxycorticosterone

11 β Hydroxylase

Corticosterone

18 Hydroxylase

Aldosterone

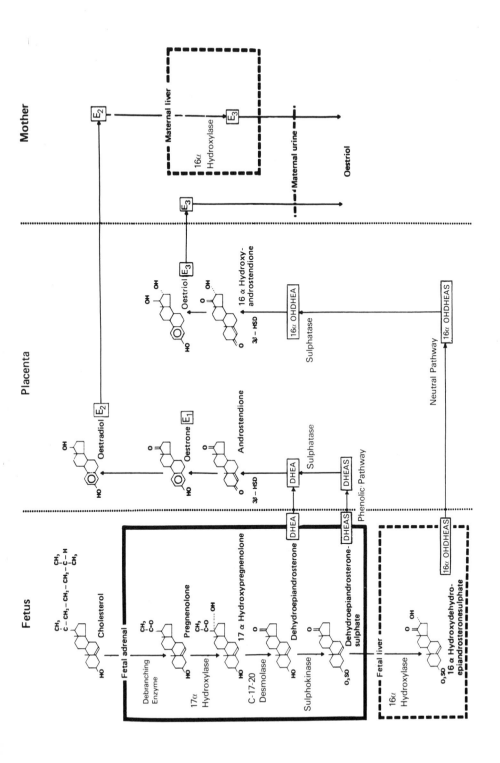

the maternal to the fetal circulation, but most of the maternal cortisol reaching the placenta is metabolized to cortisone which, though present in the fetal circulation in higher concentrations than cortisol, is without biological activity in the fetus.

The fetal adrenal: its role in determining the duration of pregnancy
Cortisol is detectable in the fetal circulation from the tenth week, and levels increase as gestation progresses, but its role in human parturition is uncertain. In the sheep a surge in fetal cortisol secretion prior to the onset of labour probably plays a vital role in initiating labour by activating placental enzymes (17 α-hydroxylase and C_{17-20} lyase) which cause a diversion of progesterone synthesis to oestrogen synthesis. The oestrogens are believed to increase synthesis of prostaglandin $F_{2\alpha}$ in the decidua and fetal membranes, the prostaglandin serving as a myometrial stimulant. If there is a surge in fetal cortisol secretion around the time of labour in the human, as is suggested by observations of amniotic fluid and umbilical arterial cortisol levels, it could be secondary to the stress of labour. There have been claims in the clinical literature that the duration of pregnancies in which fetal adrenal function is defective — as in anencephaly or congenital adrenal hypoplasia — is prolonged, but not all authorities are agreed on this; the problem of gathering reliable data is, of course, that where human pregnancies are carefully monitored, any pregnancy which looks like being over-long is not allowed to run its 'natural' course. The issue is discussed further in the next Chapter (p. 136).

The fetal adrenal: its role in preparing the fetus for extrauterine life (Fig. 7.10)
Although the role of the human fetal adrenal cortex with respect to the onset of parturition is unproven, certain other functions are more clearly established. The human fetal lung has glucocorticoid receptors which, when stimulated, activate the enzymes required for surfactant synthesis. Neonates which develop the respiratory distress syndrome have lower umbilical blood and amniotic fluid cortisol levels than those which do not. Prenatal administration of glucocorticoids to the mother enhances fetal lung maturation.

The fetal adrenal cortex promotes the deposition of glycogen in the fetal liver and fetal myocardium, causes fetal thymus regression, and activates phenylethanolamine-N-methyl transferase (PNMT) in the adrenal medulla, which is necessary for the synthesis of adrenaline from noradrenaline.

The neonatal period
After birth the adrenal cortex undergoes major structural reorganization, the fetal zone regressing completely by the end of the first month. Over the same period the definitive cortex differentiates into the three-zone structure of the adult gland, but throughout this period appears to be able to carry out its metabolic and electrolyte regulatory functions. During the neonatal period secretion of corticosterone predominates over cortisol, while aldosterone levels in the neonate rise after the 11th day, and remain elevated throughout the first year of life.

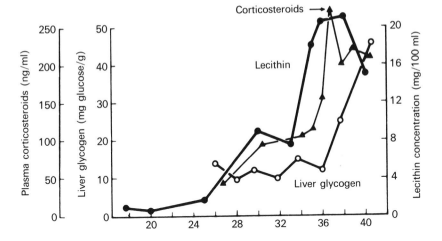

Fig. 7.10 Graph to show the relation between the concentrations of corticosteroids in fetal plasma, lecithin in amniotic fluid, and glycogen in the fetal liver during pregnancy in the human. (Copied from Biggers, J.D. (1980). In: *Medical Physiology*, vol. 2, 14th edn. Ed. by V.B. Mountcastle. C.V. Mosby, St Louis.) (From Liggins, G.C. and Rees, L. (1975). *New Zealand Medical Journal* 81, 486.)

The adrenal medulla

Cells of the human fetal adrenal medulla synthesize little or no adrenaline, the chromaffin cells producing noradrenaline almost exclusively. The extent of adrenaline synthesis depends on the activity of the enzyme, PNMT, catalysing the methylation of noradrenaline to adrenaline. Little is known of the role of the adrenal medulla in the fetus. In the neonate, adrenaline may play a part in the response to hypoglycaemia, while noradrenaline plays an important role as a sympathetic neurotransmitter which activates thermogenesis in brown adipose tissue.

Posterior pituitary hormones

Arginine vasopressin and vasotocin have been identified in the human posterior pituitary early in the second trimester. The proportion of vasotocin decreases as pregnancy advances. Oxytocin is demonstrable in umbilical cord plasma in the neonate, but its function is unclear.

The pancreas

Pancreatic α-cells appear first in the fetal human pancreas at the ninth week. β-cells appear during the 11th week. α-cells outnumber β-cells throughout fetal life, but the ratio reaches 1:1 at term, and in adult life there are between 3 and 9 times as many β-cells as α-cells.

Insulin is present in the fetus from the 11th week, and its concentration in fetal plasma rises throughout gestation. Both glucose and amino acids stimulate fetal insulin secretion. One function of fetal insulin is to promote cellular uptake of amino acids and protein synthesis; control of insulin by amino acids would therefore be appropriate. Another of insulin's functions in the fetus is the lowering of blood glucose level; this maximizes the glucose concentration gradient between mother and fetus and thereby promotes fetal uptake of glucose. The influence of high fetal blood glucose on fetal insulin secretion is apparent in fetuses of diabetic women, even if their diabetes is well controlled. The intermittent fetal hyperglycaemia which occurs in such cases causes hypertrophy and hyperplasia of the islets of Langerhans and a rise in fetal pancreatic insulin content. This hypersecretion of insulin causes an enhancement of lipogenesis, and babies born to diabetic mothers have a particularly cherubic appearance. There is normally an inverse relation between the quality of control of maternal diabetes and the degree of obesity in the offspring (Steele: *Gynaecology, Obstetrics and the Neonate*, Chapter 11). The hyperinsulinaemia may persist postnatally, causing rapid and potentially dangerous hypoglycaemia.

Glucagon is present in the fetus from the eighth week of gestation and, since the placenta is impermeable to glucagon, must arise from the fetal pancreas. In the rat chronic, but not acute, hypoglycaemia raises glucagon levels. In both rats and humans, plasma glucagon rises postnatally. Neural control of glucagon secretion may be involved in response to stress. Glucagon is probably an important component in the metabolic adjustments occurring in the postnatal period, especially for the maintenance of blood glucose levels between birth and the first feed.

Calcium-regulating hormones

Total calcium concentrations are somewhat higher in the fetus than in the mother throughout gestation, because calcium is actively transported from maternal to fetal circulation against a concentration gradient. Total plasma calcium and ionized calcium levels decline rapidly after birth, reaching their lowest levels after 48 hours and returning to values close to those seen in normal adults within about a week.

The parathyroid glands of the fetus are capable of secreting parathyroid hormone (PTH) by the end of the first trimester. PTH concentrations in human neonates are quite low, and remain so for 2 to 3 days after birth; the parathyroids are probably minimally stimulated in the fetus since circulating levels of calcium are relatively high, and are regulated by a combination of placental transport and maternal calciostatic mechanisms.

In contrast fetal concentrations of thyrocalcitonin (TCT) are quite high in the neonate and decline only slowly after birth. Neonatal hypocalcaemia may arise in part from unduly high levels of thyrocalcitonin. Vitamin D and its derivatives 25-OHD, $1,25(OH)_2D$, and $24,25(OH)_2D$ are generally present in lower concentrations in the fetus than in the mother, but being fat-soluble probably pass readily across the placenta.

Lipid metabolism

The extent of fat deposition in the fetus depends largely on the same factors that influence overall fetal growth; in particular, as already mentioned, babies born to diabetic mothers tend to form large adipose tissue deposits. Fats serve as an important source of energy to the newborn.

Fatty acid synthesis begins during the 16th week and occurs at a high rate in human fetuses; the rate of this synthesis decreases rapidly after birth. Fatty acids diffuse across the placenta, but transport mechanisms may exist, particularly for essential fatty acids. In most species, fatty acids and triglyceride concentrations in the fetal blood are lower than in the mother, but rise soon after birth, often to levels higher than those found in well-fed adults. The rise is due to a combination of a milk diet and release of fatty acids from adipose tissue. Oxidation of fatty acids is greatly enhanced after birth; when this occurs in the liver, the final products are the ketone bodies acetoacetic acid, β-hydroxybutyric acid and acetone.

In the fetus ketone bodies pass readily through the placenta, but little is known about the extent of their utilization in the fetus. In the newborn, ketone bodies may contribute significantly to the provision of tissue energy; suckling rats, for example, utilize ketones for fatty acid and sterol synthesis in nervous tissue and skin.

Blood levels of triglycerides are low in the fetuses of most species, and triglycerides cannot pass across the placenta. In the human there is a postnatal rise in blood triglycerides which is closely related to food intake. The triglycerides in the fetus contain smaller amounts of unsaturated fatty acids and a larger amount of palmitic acid than the triglycerides of the mother, indicating that most fetal fatty acids are synthesized *de novo*. After birth, the fatty acid composition is closely related to the fatty acid composition of the milk.

Phospholipids are synthesized by the fetus, and do not cross the placental barrier. They are particularly important in the development of nervous tissue, and in the lungs where they act as surfactants (see p. 106).

Brown adipose tissue: its role in neonatal thermoregulation

Adipose tissue in fetuses and neonates is of two kinds: white adipose tissue (WAT) and brown adipose tissue (BAT). The cells of BAT are irregularly shaped, have numerous mitochondria and dense cristae, and are plentifully supplied with sympathetic nerves. When activated, the tissue has a very high oxygen consumption. Brown adipose tissue is not found in all newborn mammals, but is abundant in those with poor muscular development, such as rats, rabbits and man. Though BAT is more abundant in young animals, the earlier view that it was of little importance in adults is currently being re-examined. In the newborn, BAT is distributed around the arteries of the neck, between the shoulder blades, in the mediastinum of the thorax and around the kidneys.

Brown adipose tissue serves as the body's central heating system, which is 'ignited' by noradrenaline released from sympathetic nerve endings in response to cold. Stored fat may be used as the source of energy, but glucose and fatty acids may be drawn from the circulation. The 'burners' are the mitochondria; either there is coupled oxidative phosphorylation driving otherwise useless cycles of chemical changes simply to generate heat, or alternatively the oxidative phosphorylation may be uncoupled. Transmission of the heat generated by this *non-shivering thermogenesis* is achieved via the blood which is distributed so as to keep the upper part of the spinal cord warm. This area of the spinal cord is at least partly responsible for the control of shivering, and when BAT activity is high, shivering might be suppressed. A healthy 3 kg infant has a substantial capacity to increase its heat production; the oxygen consumption rate may rise from a resting value of 6 ml/kg/min to as high as 15 ml/kg/min, and BAT could easily account for half the observed increase.

Carbohydrate metabolism

Fetal carbohydrate metabolism

The fetus has a constant and plentiful supply of glucose, whereas the newborn obtains relatively small amounts of glucose derived from lactose in the milk. Claude Bernard demonstrated in 1859 the accumulation of glycogen in the fetal liver. Other tissues such as skeletal and cardiac muscle can and do store glycogen, but only the liver can degrade glycogen to glucose in order to replenish blood glucose. The two enzymes essential for liver glycogen metabolism are *glycogen synthetase* (which catalyses the synthesis of glycogen) and *phosphorylase* which catalyses glycogenolysis. The amount of both enzymes increases in the late fetal liver, but the synthetase is present in its active 'a' form, whereas the phosphorylase is in the inactive 'b' form. Both the amounts and activity of glycogen synthetase are increased by glucocorticoids and by insulin, whereas glucagon tends to activate phosphorylase and to inactivate glycogen synthetase. The increase in adrenal cortical function towards term is particularly important in stimulating deposition of liver glycogen, but additional factors derived from the fetal pituitary or from the placenta may also be involved.

Neonatal carbohydrate metabolism: the danger of hypoglycaemia

After birth the supply of glucose via the placenta necessarily ceases, and there is a fall in the fasting blood glucose level. The neonatal pancreas responds by increasing glucagon release and decreasing insulin release. There may also be an increase in sympathetic activity. These neuro-endocrine changes raise liver cyclic AMP levels thereby depressing glycogen synthetase and activating phosphorylase. This reduces glycogen synthesis and accelerates glycogenolysis. The resulting release of glucose from the liver restores the blood glucose concentration.

Neonatal hypoglycaemia is a major preventable cause of brain damage, and hence of mental subnormality and cerebral palsy (Steele: *Gynaecology, Obstetrics and the Neonate*, Chapter 5). The normal lower limit of blood glucose is 1.7 mmol/litre; there may be no obvious signs of hypoglycaemia, however, unless levels fall below 1.1 mmol/litre, when apnoea and fits may be seen.

Neonates show relatively poor glucose tolerance, their insulin production being sluggish after oral or intravenous glucose. The newborn needs to develop methods for the synthesis of glucose from galactose, amino acids, and glycerol; synthesis of the necessary enzymes, e.g. glucose-6-phosphatase, phosphoenolpyruvate carboxykinase, and various aminotransferases, is rapid in the postnatal period, and may be hastened by hormones such as cortisol, glucagon and thyroxine. At weaning, the carbohydrate content of the diet increases; appropriate adjustments in the activities of liver enzymes are necessary. These adjustments may be needed sooner than normal in the many infants whose exposure to high carbohydrate diets is hastened by early introduction of commercial non-milk infant foods.

The premature neonate does not possess the full complement of gluconeogenic enzymes at birth and this may contribute to the hypoglycaemia which may occur in such infants. An additional factor may be inadequacy of liver glycogen stores, which are also found to be very low in low-birth-weight full-term infants dying within a few days of birth, or in infants who have used up all their glycogen in response to severe asphyxia. Postnatal hypoglycaemia is also seen in many of the heavy babies born to diabetic mothers; in these cases the hyperactivity of the β-cells which has developed in utero results in abnormally high insulin levels at birth, resulting in a sharp drop in blood glucose when the abundant maternal glucose supply ceases. There are a number of rare conditions involving genetic defects in liver carbohydrate metabolism which may also result in hypoglycaemia, or in the inability to convert hexoses such as galactose or fructose to glucose.

The central nervous system

The blood-brain barrier

In the fetus, the concentration of protein in the cerebrospinal fluid is remarkably high compared with the adult. This could indicate immaturity in the blood-brain barrier, but morphological studies indicate that the necessary tight junctions between cerebral capillary endothelial cells and between choroid plexus epithelial cells are well formed at a very early stage of fetal life. Proteins in the CSF may either (a) be transported there from blood plasma by a system of intracellular transport by choroid plexus epithelial cells, or (b) be products of developing neurons in which the presence of specific proteins may be of great developmental significance.

Brain metabolism

The most striking feature of the fetal brain is that from the 32nd week of gestation, it contains the three key enzymes necessary to oxidize ketone bodies. Moreover, the brains of infants and children between 6 weeks and 12 years have been shown to oxidize ketone bodies in vivo.

Electrophysiological activity

Sleeping for about 16 hours per day is normal in the neonate, with the sleeping time divided about equally between rapid-eye-movement sleep (REM, or 'paradoxical sleep') and quiet ('non-REM') sleep. Over the first 2 years of life, total sleep decreases to about 12 hours per day, with about three-quarters of that time being spent in quiet (non-REM) sleep. The amount of REM sleep is thus approximately halved over the first two years of postnatal life.

Drugs

Certain drugs, particularly those which are lipid-soluble, can easily cross from maternal to fetal blood. Similar considerations apply to the entry of drugs from the fetal circulation into the fetal brain. Heroin, morphine and methadone all produce withdrawal symptoms in babies. Many of the drugs used to alleviate pain during labour (e.g. pethidine) may enter the fetal brain, and depress normal postnatal (e.g. suckling) behaviour with consequences which may lead inexorably to failure of lactation and of the normal postpartum behavioural interactions between mother and infant which contribute to the successful establishment of normal maternal care.

Development of reflexes

A vast repertoire of reflex responses has been demonstrated in the developing fetus. The earliest reflexes are probably mediated by the lower parts of the central nervous system — mid-brain, hind-brain and spinal cord. These early responses (before about the 20th week of gestation) are relatively sterotyped, but later the pattern of behaviour becomes more variable and complex — presumably as the maturing cerebral cortex becomes involved in regulation.

Further reading

Assali, N.S and Brinkman, C.R. (eds)(1972). *Pathophysiology of Gestation. Vol. 2: Fetal-placental disorders.* Academic Press, New York.
Austin, C.R. and Short, R.V. (eds)(1982). *Reproduction in Mammals.* 2nd edn. Vol. 2: *Embryonic and Fetal Development.* Cambridge University Press, Cambridge.
Beard, R.W. and Nathanielsz, P.W. (eds)(1976). *Fetal Physiology and Medicine.* W.B. Saunders, London.
Cheek, D.B., Graystone, J.E. and Niall, M. (1977). Factors controlling fetal growth. *Clinics in Obstetrics and Gynecology* **20**, 925–942.
Comline, R.S., Cross, K.W., Dawes, G.S. and Nathanielsz, P.W. (eds)(1973). *Foetal and Neonatal Physiology: Proceedings of the Sir Joseph Barcroft Centenary Symposium.* Cambridge University Press, Cambridge.
Dawes, G.S. (1968). *Foetal and Neonatal Physiology.* Year Book Medical Publishers, Chicago.
Dougherty, C.R.S. and Jones, A.D. (1982). The determinants of birth weight. *American Journal of Obstetrics and Gynecology* **144**, 190–200.
Dryden, R. (1978). *Before Birth.* Heinemann, London.
Elliot, K. and Whelan, J. (eds)(1981). *The Fetus and Independent Life.* Ciba Foundation Symposium No. 86. Pitman, London.
Fairweather, D.V.I. and Eskes, T.K.A.B. (eds)(1978). *Amniotic Fluid: Research and Clinical Application.* 2nd edn. Excerpta Medica, Amsterdam.

Nathanielsz, P.W. (1976). *Fetal Endocrinology: an Experimental Approach.* North-Holland, Amsterdam.

Odell, G.B. (1980). *Neonatal Hyperbilirubinaemia.* Grune and Stratton, New York.

Stave, U. (ed.)(1978). *Perinatal Physiology.* Plenum, New York.

Tanner, J.M. (1978). *Foetus into Man.* Open Books, London.

Tulchinsky, D. and Ryan, K.J. (1980). *Maternal-Fetal Endocrinology.* W.B. Saunders, Philadelphia.

8

Parturition

Introduction

The process by which the fetus, placenta, and associated membranes are expelled from the uterus after a minimum of 26 weeks is called parturition. It is achieved by a crescendo of maternal myometrial activity, the mechanisms underlying which will now be considered. We shall begin with the functional anatomy of a normal human parturition, and will then discuss the changes occurring at a tissue level during the initiation of parturition. Finally we shall attempt to integrate the various factors which contribute to the onset of labour.

Normal parturition

During pregnancy there is a general softening and stretching of pelvic tissues, particularly of ligaments and the soft tissues of the vagina. There is also some shortening and dilatation of the cervix. The resulting relaxation permits some increase in pelvic capacity. The onset of 'true labour' is marked by the onset of regular contractions of the uterus which show a progressive increase in amplitude and frequency, and cause increasing discomfort; these properties of the contractions distinguish them from the contractions which normally occur throughout pregnancy. A second criterion for the onset of labour is a 'show' of blood and mucus from the vagina, which is associated with the dislodging of the cervical mucus plug, the blood loss being associated with the separation of fetal membranes from the uterine wall (Steele: *Gynaecology, Obstetrics and the Neonate,* Chapter 2).

The first stage of labour

The uterine contractions, the regular onset of which marks the beginning of the first stage of labour, are characterized by a pattern of activity whereby a wave of excitations normally passes downward, lasting longer in the body (fundus) of the uterus than in the lower part of the uterus; the contraction is not only longer but also more powerful in the body of the uterus, and the pattern thus shows *fundal dominance.* This pattern of activity contributes to the *effacement* of the cervix. The effectiveness of the uterine muscle in expelling the fetus depends on it being anchored by ligaments which are attached in the region of the cervix. These are the cardinal ligaments laterally, the uterosacral ligaments posteriorly, and the pubocervical ligaments anteriorly. By pulling against these ligaments, the uterus pushes the baby through the soft tissues and bony pelvis that constitute the birth canal. Descent is oscillatory: the baby descends during each contraction, but retreats somewhat during the following relaxation owing to the resistance and elasticity of the birth canal structures. The first stage of labour ends when the cervix is fully dilated. The fetal membranes may or may not rupture at some time during the first stage; if they do rupture, the amniotic fluid is discharged via the vagina.

Contractions of the abdominal musculature during the first stage of labour are counterproductive. They can cause an undue rise in intrauterine pressure which may have detrimental effects on fetal oxygenation, and stretch the central uterine supporting ligaments leading to an increased likelihood of later uterine prolapse. The duration of the first stage in primigravidae is commonly about 6 to 12 hours from the onset of regular contractions; in multigravidae the duration is shorter.

The second stage of labour

This stage lasts 15–45 minutes in multigravidae, and 45–120 minutes in primigravidae, during which the fetal head descends, and can readily be palpated. A strong 'bearing-down reflex' occurs during this stage of labour and is similar to that which comes into play during defaecation. After inspiration, the glottis is closed and the woman pushes down with the aid of her diaphragm and the muscles of her abdominal wall.

The third stage of labour

During this stage which begins after the birth of the baby, strong uterine contractions continue. They are normally painless, and result in the delivery of the placenta and fetal membranes.

Maternal physiology during labour

Hyperventilation is common during the first stage of labour and tends to result in a reduction of Pa_{CO_2}. Breath-holding during the second stage of labour tends to elevate Pa_{CO_2}. If hyperventilation during the first stage is excessive, it may result in a very low Pa_{CO_2}, with consequent reduction of maternal blood pressure, dizziness, and possible fetal asphyxia.

Arterial blood pressure during the second stage may rise by about 30 mmHg (4.0 kPa) putting the hypertensive patient at risk of cerebral haemorrhage. A combination of panting, vomiting, haemorrhage, and sweating associated with anxiety may contribute to water loss during labour.

Fetal physiology during labour

The only physiological parameters which are readily observable in the fetus during labour are the rate and rhythm of the heart. The normal range of heart rate is 120 to 160 beats per minute. This rate may fall as a result of umbilical cord compression, or stretching or pressure on the fetal head. A fall of fetal heart rate occurring *during* a contraction ('Type 1 dip') is common. However, if the heart rate falls *after* the peak of a contraction ('Type 2 dip') this is commonly associated with abnormal placental function and is regarded as more serious.

Samples of blood may be taken from the fetal scalp during labour in order to determine fetal acid-base balance. During labour fetal blood pH normally falls from 7.3 to 7.2, the reduction being associated with a depression of placental gas exchange. This reduction is more obvious during the second stage of labour when hypoxia, consequent upon the mother's pushing the baby through the birth canal, exacerbates the metabolic acidosis. Particularly dangerous is the combination of hypoxia and hyperglycaemia which can arise if the parturient mother is given glucose infusions; accumulation of lactate in both mother and fetus can cause damage to the fetal brain.

Changes in tissues

Myometrium

Parturition depends upon coordination of the contraction of the smooth muscle of the uterus with involuntary contraction of the striated muscle of the abdominal wall, and increasing compliance of the connective tissue of the cervix. The contraction of the uterus must, in order to be effective, involve almost simultaneous activation of adequately developed myometrial cells; thus growth, excitation, and propagation must all be considered.

Excitation of smooth muscle depends on alterations in the membrane potential of the smooth muscle cell. If the membrane potential is small (i.e. about -35 mV) the membrane enters a refractory state and is incapable of generating action potentials because of inactivation of the sodium channels which must open to cause the rising phase of the action potential. Myometrial cells of immature animals are in just such a depolarized state, and this accounts for their inactivity. Conversely if the membrane potential is very large (hyperpolarized), it becomes difficult for electrical, mechanical or chemical stimuli to depolarize the membrane to the threshold potential required for the generation of action potentials; this hyperpolarized state arises in myometrium exposed to progesterone, which increases potassium permeability and thus increases membrane potential. If it is to become active and responsive, the membrane must therefore be adequately, but not excessively, polarized (i.e. to about -50 mV); such a state is achieved by exposure to oestrogens, whereupon slow fluctuations in membrane potential (*pacemaker potentials*) cause bursts of superimposed action potentials. These 'spikes' cause a sharp increase in intracellular Ca^{2+} concentration, partly as a result of influx from extracellular fluid, and partly by liberation of Ca^{2+} bound in the sparse sarcoplasmic reticulum in the vesicles which are closely applied to the inner surface of the plasma membrane; contraction is thereby initiated.

There are at least two possible mechanisms for propagation of activity in the uterus. Since the myometrial cells lie in series with other cells, then contraction in one cell will cause stretching of its neighbours; this will in turn depolarize the membrane of the stretched cell, thereby initiating action potentials and contraction in it. But there is also evidence for direct electrical coupling between neighbouring cells, occurring at gap junctions (nexuses) which form low-resistance contacts between cells; we do not know what factors control their development, but it is presumed to be under hormonal control. An oestrogen-primed uterus which is under the influence of progesterone propagates electrical activity rather poorly; the propagation improves upon the withdrawal of progesterone. Oestrogens also act on myometrium in other ways: they stimulate synthesis of muscle proteins, and markedly enhance myometrial blood flow.

Cervical connective tissue

Connective tissue plays an important part in retaining the conceptus within the uterus during pregnancy. The proportion of connective tissue increases from the body of the uterus (where 70 per cent of the tissue is smooth muscle) to the lower part of the body of the cervix (which has just 6 per cent of smooth muscle). During most of pregnancy the connective tissue resists stretch, permitting slow distension of the body of the uterus but maintaining closure of the cervix. Towards the end of pregnancy, the compliance of the collagenous connective tissue increases permitting expansion of the lower part of the uterus — thus allowing the fetus to descend into the pelvic inlet. Eventually the cervix changes from a firm indistensible structure to become soft, yielding and compliant. How do these changes come about?

Collagen is made up of helical strands of amino acids bound together to form fibrils. Between these fibrils is a matrix composed of glycosaminoglycans (mucopolysaccharides) which include hyaluronate chondroitin sulphate, dermatan sulphate and keratan sulphate. The proportion of glycosaminoglycans and water postpartum is greater than in the nonpregnant cervix; the increase is largely due to an increase in the amount of keratan sulphate which does not bind to collagen and could thus be responsible for loosening collagen bundles and increasing the compliance of the cervix. We do not know how this alteration in cervical compliance is controlled. In some species an ovarian hormone, relaxin, may be involved, but it is not particularly important in women. Elevated oestrogen concentration during pregnancy may contribute. Prostaglandins can produce changes in the cervix characteristic of those occurring at parturition, and small doses of prostaglandins administered intravaginally cause effacement and increase compliance of the 'clinically unfavourable' cervix.

Control of uterine activity

The increase in uterine activity at the end of pregnancy is brought about by the interplay of a variety of factors. It was thought that the primary cause was the withdrawal of progesterone from myometrium at the end of pregnancy. Progesterone is needed for the maintenance of pregnancy and is synthesized by the human placenta. Despite compelling evidence that progesterone withdrawal can precipitate parturition in species which depend on the corpus luteum as a source of progesterone throughout pregnancy (e.g. rabbit and

134 Parturition

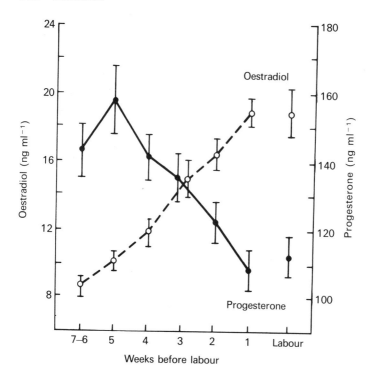

Fig. 8.1 The results of a study of Turnbull and others (1974) showing mean ±SEM levels of plasma progesterone and oestradiol in 33 primigravidae during the seven weeks before the spontaneous onset of labour and in the second stage of labour. The fall of progesterone level during the last weeks of pregnancy is clear in this study, but some authorities remain sceptical. (Turnbull, A.C., Flint, A.P.F., Jeremy, J.Y., Patten, P.T., Keirse, M.J.N.C. and Anderson, A.B.M. (1974). *Lancet* i, 101.)

goat), it is difficult to maintain the view that it can account for the onset of parturition in women. Plasma progesterone concentrations probably do not fall markedly until after delivery of the placenta, though some eminent authorities dispute this (see Figs 6.6 and 8.1); furthermore, administration of progestagens to pregnant women does not delay labour. In the light of this contrary evidence, variations on the 'progesterone withdrawal theory' for the onset of labour have been proposed. According to one view, a progesterone-binding protein appears in fetal membranes late in pregnancy; this would compete for progesterone with other sites and lead, in effect, to local progesterone withdrawal. Alternatively it is suggested that the placenta, being the major source of progesterone, could exert a local blockage of myometrium activity; according to this view, the myometrium overlying the placenta will be bathed in fluid in which concentrations of steroids bear little relation to those in peripheral maternal plasma. The fact is, however, that no good evidence exists to show that myometrial concentrations fail to reflect peripheral plasmal concentrations, and it must be assumed that progesterone withdrawal cannot account for the onset of human labour.

If, then, labour in the woman is not triggered by removal of inhibition, we should direct our attention to agents which stimulate uterine activity. These include mechanical stretch, oestrogens, oxytocin, and prostaglandins. Prostaglandins are now believed to play a central role in parturition. Those capable of acting on uterine muscle at the end of pregnancy are probably synthesized in the human endometrium, since this tissue contains quite high concentrations of prostaglandins which fall at the start of pregnancy, suggesting that their synthesis is inhibited by the presence of the developing conceptus. Decidual tissue contains an active prostaglandin (PG) synthetase, but myometrium, cervix, placenta and fetal membranes may also contribute to PG synthesis.

Synthesis of PG is dependent on the provision of the precursor, arachidonic acid, which is stored in an esterified form in cells, being released when the enzyme phospholipase A_2 acts on stored glycerophospholipids. This enzyme is present in an inactive membrane-bound form in lysosomes of decidual and fetal membranes, and is activated when the stability of the lysosomal membrane is changed. Towards the end of pregnancy, arachidonic acid is incorporated into phospholipid stores in decidua and fetal membranes, a process which is thought to be enhanced by progesterone (Fig. 8.2).

The release of this stored arachidonic acid by destabilization of lysosomal membranes may be the direct effect of rising oestrogen levels at the end of pregnancy, but could result from the stimulation by oestrogens of the formation of oxytocin receptors; thus oxytocin, without any change in its plasma concentration, could increase PG release.

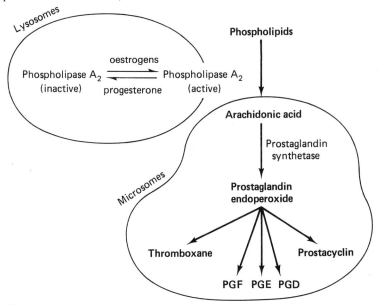

Fig. 8.2 Pathway for biosynthesis of primary prostaglandins, thromboxane and prostacyclins. The arachidonic acid 'cascade' is shown in bold letters and bold arrows. The main rate-limiting step is the activation of phospholipase A, shown at the top left of the diagram. (From Liggins, G.C. (1979). *British Medical Bulletin* **35**, 145–150.)

The timing of parturition

The dominant role of the fetus in the sheep

In the sheep the fetus has been shown to play a dominant role in determining the time of initiation of parturition. The initial observation was that the weed *Veratrum californicum*, consumed by pregnant ewes, caused developmental abnormalities of the head in the fetal lamb resulting in the absence of the pituitary gland. This resulted in the prolongation of pregnancy for many weeks, which could be mimicked by hypophysectomy or bilateral adrenalectomy of the fetus. Adrenocorticotrophic hormone infusion into fetal lambs, on the other hand, resulted in premature delivery. Parturition in the sheep is now thought to be triggered by a sharp increase in cortisol concentration in the fetal circulation, which induces activity in the placenta of enzymes such as 17 α-hydroxylase and C_{17-20} lyase, the effect of which is to direct placental progesterone to synthesis of oestrogens. Progesterone secretion falls, oestradiol secretion rises, and the synthesis and release of $PGF_{2\alpha}$ is stimulated. The increase in fetal cortisol seems to be due mainly to enhanced sensitivity of the fetal adrenal cortex to ACTH.

Control in the human

The role of the fetus

Matters are not as clear-cut in the human. Obviously most forms of experiment are impossible, and data from clinical studies do not support the view that parturition is controlled by mechanisms analogous to those described for the sheep. Despite earlier claims, it now seems that pituitary or adrenal hypoplasia is compatible with spontaneous onset of labour. Mean gestation length is unaffected in pregnancies involving anencephalic fetuses, if such pregnancies are uncomplicated by polyhydramnios. The human placenta lacks steroid 17 α-hydroxylase, and so, even though cortisol levels in the fetal circulation normally rise during the last month of pregnancy, no diversion of progesterone into oestrogen synthesis can occur in the placenta. The major substrate for placental oestrogen synthesis later in pregnancy is the androgen — dehydroepiandrosterone sulphate — secreted by the *fetal zone* of the fetal adrenal cortex. But placental oestrogen synthesis is probably not an essential prerequisite for parturition because pregnant women treated with corticosteroids which depress both androgen and oestrogen production by the feto-placental unit go into spontaneous labour at the usual time. The crucial alterations in tissue function that initiate human parturition may take place not in the fetus, but rather in the chorion (i.e. trophoblast and underlying fetal mesenchyme), both placental and extraplacental. This proposition is consistent with the observations that (a) human patients enter labour about one week after fetal death in utero, and (b) the birth of human twins in a double uterus may be separated by days or even weeks.

Other controlling influences

It is important to distinguish between (a) the control of the onset of parturition which is poorly understood, and (b) the fine timing and regulation of the course of labour, once initiated. Many animals choose a dark quiet place for parturition. In mice an unfamiliar disturbing environment (a goldfish bowl) delays the onset and duration of parturition. There is a weak 24-hour rhythmicity in the timing of the onset of labour in women, with labour tending to begin in the early hours of the morning.

It may be that endogenous *oxytocin* (the word, appropriately, is derived from the Greek meaning 'quick birth') is important in expediting, if not initiating, labour. The concentration of oxytocin in maternal plasma is low during the first stage of human labour, but is sometimes higher during the second stage. Oxytocin release is inhibited by stress. The reduction of emotional stress before and during parturition is a major objective of many 'natural childbirth' techniques, and they may owe their effectiveness to the creation of optimum conditions for the operation of the 'fetus-ejection reflex', whereby mechanical stimulation of uterus, cervix and vagina will promote oxytocin release.

Shepherds, stud grooms and herdsmen know the importance of providing quiet, peaceful and reasonably familiar surroundings for pregnant animals prior to parturition. Sheep, horses and cows are presumably less anxious about impending parturition than many women; therefore, in view of what we know about the inhibitory effects of emotional stress and apprehension on uterine activity, efforts to provide a stress-free environment for women in labour should be encouraged. Simple humane steps to minimize the fear of parturition (such as the unbroken presence of a reassuring caretaker during labour, and the provision of an environment resembling a familiar bedroom) could do much to obviate the need for heroic obstetrical measures to cope with situations such as uterine inertia whose occurrence, in some cases at least, might have been avoided by tender loving care.

Summary

Parturition is a 'cascade phenomenon', comprising a number of processes which interact in a positive-feedback manner so that, once initiated, parturition normally proceeds to an expeditious conclusion. The list of the main ingredients which constitute the process is largely established, consisting of prostaglandins, oestrogens, falling progesterone levels, oxytocin, the fetal adrenal, the external environment, and mechanical stretch of the uterus, with possible contributions from the uterine autonomic innervation and from relaxin. What is less clear is the precise causal chain of events. The impossibility of experimental interference with human parturition makes it likely that this uncertainty will remain.

Further reading

Ciba Foundation Symposium No. 47 (1977). *The Fetus and Birth.* Elsevier/Excerpta Medica/North-Holland, Amsterdam.

Ellwood, D.A. and Anderson, A.B.M. (eds)(1981). *The Cervix in Pregnancy and Labour: Clinical and Biochemical Investigations.* Churchill Livingstone, Edinburgh.

Finn, C.A. and Porter, D.G. (1975). *The Uterus.* Elek Science, London.

Kitzinger, S. and Davis, J.A. (eds)(1978). *The Place of Birth: A study of the environment in which birth takes place with special reference to home confinements.* Oxford University Press, Oxford.

Liggins, G.C. (1979). What factors initiate labor? *Contemporary Obstetrics Gynecology* **13**, 147.

Turnbull, A.C., Flint, A.P.F., Jeremy, J.Y., Patten, P.T., Keirse, M.J.N.C. and Anderson, A:B.M. (1974). Significant fall in progesterone and rise in oestradiol levels in human peripheral plasma before onset of labour. *Lancet* **i**, 101–104.

9

Lactation and maternal behaviour

Lactation

Introduction

Lactation is all too often consigned to a few paragraphs at the end of chapters in physiology textbooks. There are a number of reasons why the mammary gland deserves more attention (Steele: *Gynaecology, Obstetrics and the Neonate*, Chapters 3, 6 and 7).

1. Breast milk is the best food for babies, and makes a major contribution to their healthy development. Recent research has refined and reinforced our understanding of the many constituents of fresh human milk which prevent disease.

2. It is a very active site of synthetic, secretory and transport mechanisms.

3. It is a major consumer, and a major provider, of metabolic energy.

4. It is a target for the action of many hormones; their effects include growth, secretion, milk ejection, and vasoconstriction.

5. It is the site of the suckling stimulus which, acting on the brain, has important endocrine and behavioural consequences; these include the suppression of the release of gonadotrophic hormones (a major contribution to the limitation of the growth of world population) and, in many women, a subjectively pleasurable sensation.

6. It is widely used in the study of the control of growth, particularly its hormonal control; not the least of the reasons is that the mammary gland is the most common site of cancer in women.

7. Human lactation has major economic repurcussions. A society in which few women breast-feed needs to manufacture or to import huge quantities of artificial infant feeding materials, with economic consequences that may be ruinous.

8. Breast feeding encourages the establishment of normal psychosocial interaction between mother and baby.

The growth and structure of the mammary gland

Postnatal development
Both male and female human babies are born with mammary glands which

have been stimulated by hormones in the fetal circulation, and their alveolar secretory cells experience withdrawal of sex steroids at birth allowing prolactin to stimulate milk secretion which reaches its maximum production 4–7 days postpartum; accordingly fluid known as 'witches' milk', with a composition similar to that of *colostrum* (see Table 9.1), can be expressed from the nipple of infants of either sex. This secretory activity subsides within the first month and the alveoli regress leaving only ducts which grow slowly prior to puberty.

Puberty

With the onset of puberty, breast growth occurs at a rate different from that of the body as a whole (*allometric* growth). Early in puberty, breast development is stimulated predominantly by oestrogens which cause elevation of the nipples, duct proliferation, increase in volume and elasticity of periductal connective tissues, enhanced vascularization and fat deposition. Later in puberty, under the combined influence of progesterone and oestrogens, lobular-alveolar development occurs. Some mammary growth is observed around puberty in many boys. This *gynaecomastia* is associated with temporary disturbances in sex steroid metabolism occurring at the time.

Adult structure

The mature breast shows a characteristic ductule-lobule-alveolar structure, the process of maturation involving stimulation by both oestrogens and progesterone supplemented by the effects of other hormones such as insulin, cortisol, thyroxine, growth hormone and prolactin. The breast is dome-shaped with the *areola* — a circular pigmented area — located in its centre. There are large variations in the form, size and location of breasts.

Small ducts from large sebaceous glands (*Montgomery's glands*) open into the peripheral area of the areola; these glands enlarge during pregnancy and lactation and secrete a milky fluid which serves to lubricate the areola and nipple. The mammary ducts in the breast of the nonpregnant woman consist of a simple two-layered epithelium. In the alveoli there are basal cells with a clear cytoplasm, darkly staining eosinophilic cells found in the lumen of the alveoli, and myoepithelial cells which lie close to basement membrane. There are periodic changes in the mammary glands associated with the menstrual cycle. In the days prior to menstruation, water retention leads to relatively large breast volume and some enlargement of the lumen of alveoli which contain secretory material; thus heavy tender breasts may be characteristic of the premenstrual period. After menstruation there is degeneration of some glandular cells, reduction in lobular-alveolar size, and disappearance of tissue interstitial fluid. As a result the breasts reach their smallest about a week after the onset of menstruation.

The *blood supply* is provided mainly by the internal mammary artery and the lateral thoracic artery, and there is both deep and superficial venous drainage. The extensive *lymphatic drainage* of the breast is particularly important because about 5 per cent of women suffer from breast cancer at some time in their life. Malignant cells can be widely distributed by the lymphatics.

The mammary gland is *innervated* by both somatic afferent and autonomic efferent nerves. Myoepithelial cells lack innervation, and glandular cells have at most sparse innervation. The autonomic innervation is exclusively from unmyelinated postganglionic sympathetic nerves which cause contraction of the smooth muscle of the nipple, areola (and thus nipple erection), and of the vascular smooth muscle (and thus vasoconstriction). The sensory innervation of the peripheral skin of the breast is like that of hairy skin in other parts of the body. The superficial epidermis of the nipple and areola is poorly innervated; light touch is not well perceived. There are, however, a large number of deeper dermal receptors which contribute to the mechanical sensitivity of the nipple and areola, which is the basis of (a) the afferent limb of reflex arcs which cause release of prolactin and oxytocin, and (b) the pleasureable sensation which may accompany mechanical stimulation of the region. After puberty, the tactile sensitivity of all areas of women's breasts is greater than that of men's breasts. Tactile sensitivity of women's breasts varies with the menstrual cycle, being greatest at mid-cycle and at menstruation. A marked increase in breast sensitivity occurs within 24 hours after parturition which could facilitate the suckling-induced release of oxytocin and prolactin.

Growth during pregnancy
The increasing levels of oestrogens and progesterone produce striking changes in the breasts. At an early stage, cutaneous blood vessels become more prominent. The nipples enlarge and become more erect, while the tissue behind the nipple loosens permitting it to be more readily pulled outward during suckling. The areolae enlarge, and Montgomery's glands increase in size. There is intense sprouting and branching of ducts, and lobules of secretory tissue grow by invading and replacing adipose tissue, this glandular growth accounts for the increase in breast size seen in the last 6 months of pregnancy. Mammary blood flow and interstitial fluid both rise within the first month of gestation and the breasts become increasingly firm and sensitive. A straw-coloured nipple discharge which may occur at this time probably arises from transudation of plasma into the duct system. By term each breast has increased markedly in weight and subcutaneous veins are dilated — blood flow being almost twice that in the nonpregnant state. The ducts and alveoli dilate, becoming partly filled with colostrum. Mammary epithelial proliferation tends to decline around midpregnancy; at this time alveolar epithelial stem cells differentiate under the influence of prolactin, progesterone, hPL, and other metabolic hormones such as insulin and corticosteroids, to assume either a contractile function as myoepithelial cells, or a secretory function.

The DNA and RNA content of the alveolar epithelial cells increases, and intracytoplasmic fat droplets accumulate. Lymphocytes appear in connective tissue surrounding the alveoli; these are probably plasma cells derived from Peyer's patches in the intestine which have migrated via mediastinal lymph nodes and the circulation and have 'homed in' on the mammary gland where they will produce the secretory IgA in milk.

The events described above prepare the breasts of the pregnant woman for lactation, and the volume of milk secreted during the *puerperium* (the period immediately after parturition) is closely related to the extent of mammary glandular development during pregnancy.

The onset of milk secretion (*lactogenesis*) occurs during pregnancy; however, although from midpregnancy mammary alveolar cells are actively synthesizing milk fat and proteins, only small amounts are released into the lumen. The development of this functional capacity of the secretory cells develops as a result of the changing levels of hormones in the maternal circulation, but it is only with the withdrawal of the hormones of pregnancy — notably progesterone but possibly also hPL — that prolactin becomes able to stimulate the synthesis and secretion of milk into the alveoli. Prior to this, some *colostrum* is secreted into the mammary alveoli and can be expelled from the nipples; it is composed of water, minerals, fat droplets, round cells (lymphocytes, monocytes and histiocytes), and 'Donne bodies', which are a coagulation of round cells and desquamated phagocytic alveolar cells.

Lactogenesis (Fig. 9.1.)

Lactogenesis — the initiation of a copious flow of milk at or about the time of parturition — is accompanied by changes in the structure and function of mammary secretory cells. There is rapid growth of the endoplasmic reticulum and Golgi apparatus. The RNA : DNA ratio, an index of the cellular potential for protein synthesis, increases, as does the activity of many enzymes.

Lactogenesis is under hormonal control. The endocrine requirements can be studied in vivo in the animal deprived of its pituitary and other glands, or in vitro by observing mammary tissue in culture. Such studies have demonstrated the necessity for cortisol, insulin and prolactin for lactogenesis; these hormones can thus be regarded as 'go' stimuli for lactation. But lactogenesis also results from a release from the inhibitory effects of steroid hormones, notably progesterone; progesterone inhibits lactogenesis, and oestrogens may also have an inhibitory effect. Progesterone acts specifically to suppress the synthesis of lactose in the mammary gland. The enzyme lactose synthetase consists of two components: one of these (galactosyl transferase) normally utilizes N-acetylglucosamine as a substrate, but in the presence of the second component, the milk protein α-lactalbumin, the substrate specificity of the galactosyl transferase is altered, so that it will catalyse the following reaction:

$$\text{UDP galactose} + \text{glucose} \rightarrow \text{lactose} + \text{UDP}$$

The role, then, of α-lactalbumin is to serve as a 'specifier protein' Alpha-lactalbumin synthesis is stimulated by insulin, cortisol and prolactin, but is inhibited by progesterone, and a rapid rise occurs in its concentration in mammary tissue at parturition when progesterone levels fall, resulting in a rise in lactose synthesis.

Plasma prolactin levels rise strikingly and steadily throughout pregnancy (see Fig. 6.4), though there is a great deal of individual variation among women in terms of the peak levels achieved. This increase in prolactin levels results from the elevated oestrogen production during pregnancy; the oestrogens act directly upon the pituitary to promote prolactin release. Progesterone decreases the release of prolactin; the rise in oestrogen:

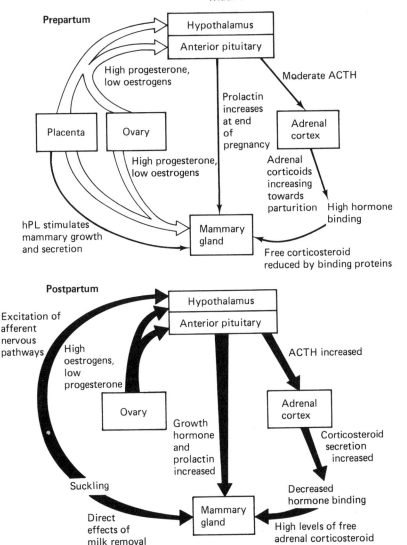

Fig. 9.1 Diagrams illustrating the control of the mammary gland prepartum and postpartum, emphasizing the factors responsible for lactogenesis.

progesterone ratio in the maternal circulation towards the end of pregnancy therefore enhances not only the lactogenic response to prolactin, but also the release of that hormone. The effects of oestrogens are not, however, exclusively stimulatory to lactogenesis; in high concentrations, oestrogens act directly on mammary tissue to inhibit its response to prolactin. After parturition, levels of both progesterone and oestrogens fall, removing the inhibition of tissue responsiveness to lactogenic hormones. Prolactin also falls after parturition in women who do not breast feed, but the suckling stimulus stimulates prolactin release causing it to attain very high levels in the early months of lactation. The presence, or just the smell, of offspring may be enough to elicit prolactin release in animals. The necessity for prolactin in lactogenesis is demonstrated by the prevention of the initiation of milk secretion after parturition in women treated with the dopamine-agonist bromocriptine, which inhibits pituitary prolactin release.

Cortisol-binding globulin (CBG) more than doubles in concentration during pregnancy, and this is associated with a rise in maternal plasma cortisol levels, in spite of a decrease in cortisol production rate. A fall in the level of CBG at the time of parturition would lead to a rise in free cortisol concentration, which may contribute to lactogenesis.

Galactopoiesis

Galactopoiesis — the maintenance of established lactation — depends on suckling by the infant, which results both in the removal of milk, and in the stimulation of the release of hormones which promote milk secretion. The removal of milk is essential for the maintenance of milk secretion. Failure of milk secretion following failure of milk removal is often attributed simply to engorgement of the alveoli and ducts with milk, resulting in compression of capillary blood vessels. But there is now evidence that a more subtle local chemical regulation of milk secretion is also present. Milk, and in particular certain fatty acids contained in it, interferes with the activation of acetyl-CoA-carboxylase, thus producing a marked inhibition of fatty acid synthesis in mammary tissue extracts. As a result of this and other local negative-feedback mechanisms, mammary tissue is able to match milk secretion to demand. Mammary glands at the time of parturition have the potential for a high level of milk secretion, but this potential may rapidly be lost — probably as a result of involution of secretory epithelium — if early demand for milk is diminished (Fig. 9.2.). The effect of demand on the secretory tissue is due both to the direct effect of the removal of milk, and to the effects of the suckling stimulus on prolactin secretion.

Milk ejection

Suckling is a potent stimulus to the release of oxytocin from the neurohypophysis (Fig. 9.3.). Oxytocin causes the contraction of myoepithelial cells which envelop the alveoli, and displaces milk from the alveoli into the larger lactiferous ducts and sinuses, from which it can readily be removed by suckling. Milk ejection (and thus presumably oxytocin release) is also stimulated by stimuli such as the sight or sound of a baby, or even the thought of nursing. Emotional stress or anxiety can inhibit milk-ejection; inhibition arises in part from centrally-mediated inhibition of the *release* of oxytocin, but the *action* of oxytocin on myoepithelial cells may also be decreased in two ways: (a) sympathetic vasoconstrictor fibres to the breast may be activated, causing constriction of blood vessels and thereby decreasing the access of circulating oxytocin to its target tissue; and (b) adrenaline and noradrenaline released during stress may exert a direct inhibitory effect on the responsiveness of myoepithelial cells to oxytocin.

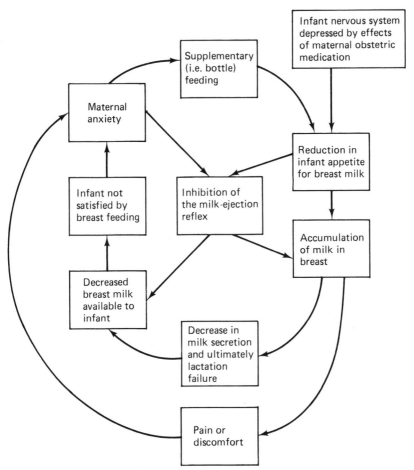

Fig. 9.2 Some causes of lactation failure. Note how depression of the appetite of the infant can lead to the establishment of a vicious circle which can end in lactation failure.

Myoepithelial cells invest the alveolar secretory epithelium, and also lie within the walls of small mammary ducts where they are arranged longitudinally. By contracting, they tend to shorten and widen the ducts thereby decreasing their resistance to the flow of milk (Fig 9.4.). Myoepithelial cells contract not only in response to oxytocin, but also when mechanically stimulated; massage of the breast by the suckling infant may therefore assist in the expulsion of some alveolar milk even in the absence of oxytocin release.

The synthesis and secretion of the components of milk

Protein

Mammary secretory epithelial cells have a well developed rough endoplasmic reticulum (RER)(Fig. 9.5.). Here the major milk proteins are synthesized before being discharged into the cavities of the RER. They are transported to the Golgi apparatus and here become condensed into microscopically visible secretory granules which move in swollen Golgi vesicles towards the cellular

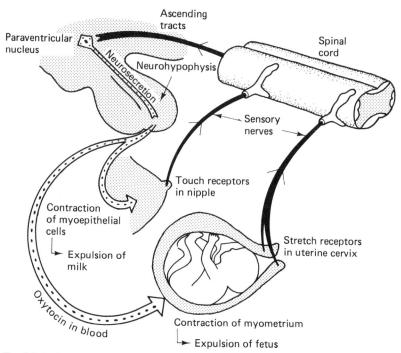

Ascending tracts

Paraventricular nucleus

Spinal cord

Neurosecretion

Neurohypophysis

Sensory nerves

Touch receptors in nipple

Contraction of myoepithelial cells

↳ Expulsion of milk

Stretch receptors in uterine cervix

Oxytocin in blood

Contraction of myometrium

↳ Expulsion of fetus

Fig. 9.3 Pathways involved in the release of oxytocin in response to suckling (the milk-ejection reflex) and distension of the birth canal (the 'fetus-ejection reflex'). Not shown are the poorly-understood, but important, pathways whereby stress can inhibit the release of oxytocin, and learned stimuli (e.g. a crying baby) can stimulate release. (From Hardy, R.N. (1981). *Endocrine Physiology*. Edward Arnold, London.)

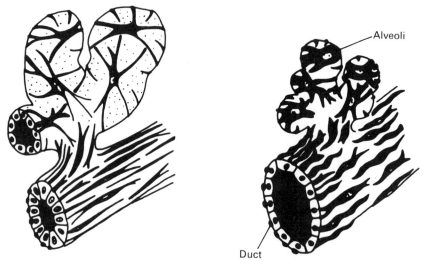

Alveoli

Duct

Fig. 9.4 The action of myoepithelial cells: as they contract they compress the secretory alveoli and shorten and widen the ducts. (From Mepham, B. (1976). *The Secretion of Milk*. Edward Arnold, London.) (Reproduced by courtesy of J.L. Linzell)

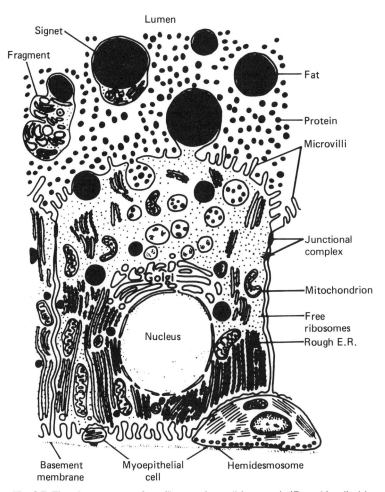

Fig. 9.5 The ultrastructure of a milk-secreting cell (see text). (From Linzell, J.L. and Peaker. M. (1971). *Physiological Reviews* **51**, 564–597.)

apex. These vesicles discharge their contents into the lumen by exocytosis.

The dominant milk immunoglobulin is secretory IgA. Lymphocytes secreting sIgA become incorporated in mammary alveolar epithelium, and some pass directly into secreted colostrum and milk.

Lactose

Alpha-lactalbumin is a major protein constituent of milk, but also serves as a 'specifier protein' (see p. 142) which enables galactosyltransferase to utilize glucose as a substrate for lactose synthesis. Lactose accumulates within the Golgi vesicles which swell with water (Fig. 9.6.) drawn in by the osmotic effect of the accumulation of lactose and proteins. Fusion of these vesicles with the apical membrane of the cell results in the extrusion of their contents into the alveolar lumen.

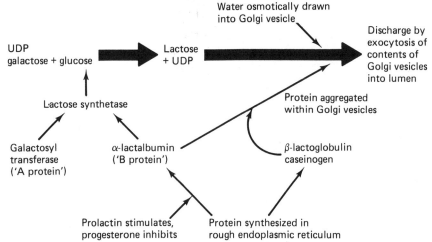

Fig. 9.6 A diagram illustrating the interdependence of the processes involved in the secretion of protein, lactose and water.

Fat

The lipids in milk are thought to be synthesized mainly in the RER of the secretory cell. *De novo* synthesis of short-chain fatty acids via the malonyl-CoA pathway requires NADPH, which is supplied mainly from the pentose cycle; the carbon in these short-chain fatty acids is derived principally from plasma glucose. The long-chain fatty acids of human milk fat are derived from plasma, i.e. from circulating free fatty acids, or from circulating triglycerides found in chylomicra or lipoproteins. Glycerol required for milk triglycerides is partly derived from hydrolyzed plasma lipids, partly by synthesis from glucose, and to a small extent from free plasma glycerol. Within the secretory cell, the lipids coalesce into increasingly large fat droplets. At the apex, each droplet is enveloped in membrane, bulges from the cell surface, and is released into the alveolar lumen (see Fig. 9.5).

Sodium and potassium

Mature milk has relatively high potassium and low sodium concentrations, indicating that these ions are probably derived from intracellular fluid. The high intracellular potassium and low intracellular sodium concentrations within the mammary secretory cell are maintained by the operation of the sodium pump with which the enzyme Na^+-K^+ *activated ATPase* is intimately associated. This enzyme is present only at the basal and lateral membranes and is absent at the apical surface of the cell. Tight junctions between neighbouring alveolar secretory cells normally impede leakage of extracellular fluid, and a rise in milk sodium concentration indicates a breakdown in these intercellular junctions. Sodium, potassium and chloride enter the milk by diffusing across the membrane down their respective electrochemical gradients. The ratios of Na^+ to K^+ concentration in mammary cells and in milk are identical, though the actual concentrations of the ions in milk are lower, because lactose accounts for about half the osmotic activity of milk which is invariably isotonic with plasma.

Other ions

Chloride ions diffuse passively from intracellular fluid into milk. Ca^{2+}, Mg^{2+}, and $PO_4{}^{3-}$ are all present in milk in concentrations exceeding those in plasma, so that active transport is probably involved in their secretion, though binding of these ions to proteins may partly account for their higher concentration in milk. Iron is bound specifically to the minor milk protein *lactoferrin*.

Water

More than 80 per cent of the weight of milk is water, and the tonicity of milk is the same as that of plasma. Water is drawn into Golgi vesicles along with the lactose synthesized with them (Fig. 9.6). The movement of water from the cytoplasm of the secretory cells into the alveolar lumen is largely governed by the osmotic effect of lactose, and of Na^+, K^+, and Cl^-—the sum of the concentration of the three ions being inversely related to that of lactose.

Other constituents

Some vitamins, e.g. B_1, B_2 and C, are present in milk in higher concentrations than in blood plasma indicating the existence of active transport mechanisms.

The composition of milk, and its implications (Table 9.1.)

The first milk to be produced in the course of lactation is *colostrum* which contains more protein, less fat, more sodium and more chloride than mature milk. The higher sodium content indicates that it is formed by a process during which there is some breakdown of the tight junctions between neighbouring alveolar secretory cells. Colostrum is a lemon-yellow viscous fluid, particularly rich in antibodies, especially secretory IgA, and various kinds of white blood cell which are phagocytic and secrete anti-bacterial agents.

Mature human milk varies between individual mothers in both composition and volume and there are 24-hour variations in secretion rate and, particularly, fat content. The volume output per day may be between 100–1100 ml. Milk fat composition varies with maternal diet and body stores. The fat composition of human milk rises three-fold as the evacuation of the mammary gland proceeds because of adsorption of fat to epithelia; thus successful milk ejection is important if the full calorific value of milk is to be obtained.

Caseins, which are phosphoproteins which readily precipitate at acid pH, form a smaller proportion of human than of cows' milk. The *curd* formed by the precipitation of human milk casein in the stomach is soft and flocculent and contrasts with the tough rubbery curd formed by cows' milk. Casein molecules are associated together in combination with calcium ion, magnesium ion, and phosphate, and milk may therefore contain much more of these ions than are present in simple aqueous solution. The *whey* proteins are those not precipitated at acid pH; they form a larger proportion of human milk protein, which is richer in lactoferrin, lysozyme and secretory IgA than is cows' milk, but contains no β-lactoglobulin and much less IgG. Lactoferrin

Table 9.1 The approximate concentration of the more important components per 100 ml of whole milk unless otherwise stated. The rate of secretion of human milk varies according to the time of day and the stage of lactation; an average of one series of measurements on the seventh day of lactation was about 400 ml in 24 hours. The fat content of milk rises as evacuation of the gland proceeds in a given nursing episode; this results from the adsorption of fat to secretory and duct surfaces

	Human colostrum	Human mature milk	Cows' milk
Water, g	–	88	88
Lactose, g	5.3	6.8	5.0
Protein, g	2.7	1.2	3.3
Casein: lactalbumin ratio	–	1:2	3:1
Fat,* g	2.9	3.8	3.7
Sodium, mg	92	15	58
Potassium, mg	66	55	138
Chloride, mg	117	43	103
Calcium, mg	31	33	125
Magnesium, mg	4	4	12
Phosphorus, mg	14	15	100
Iron, mg	0.09	0.15	0.10
Vit A, μg	89	53	34
Vit, D, μg	–	0.03	0.06
Thiamine, μg	15	16	42
Riboflavine, μg	30	43	157
Nicotinic acid, μg	75	172	85
Ascorbic acid, mg	4.4	4.3	1.6

*of which linoleic acid makes up 8.3 per cent in human mature milk and 1.6 per cent in cows' milk.

binds iron, thereby making it less available for intestinal micro-organisms. *Lysozyme (muramidase)* is a bacteriolytic enzyme present in lacrymal secretion and in breast milk; it is not destroyed in the intestines. Secretory IgA, though present in especially high concentrations in colostrum, continues to be present in breast milk for several months and is resistant to the proteolytic enzymes and low pH within the stomach. Secretory IgA acts within the gastrointestinal tract, particularly against pathogenic *Escherichia coli*, enteroviruses such as polio virus, and rotaviruses which are recently recognized pathogens causing gastroenteritis.

The disaccharide lactose, in which galactose is linked to the 4-position of glucose, accounts for almost all the carbohydrate in human milk. In the animal kingdom it is found only in mammalian milk, although it does occur in some plants. The lactose content of human milk is high compared with that of all other species. It enhances calcium absorption, provides a source of galactose (which is a necessary component of galactolipids, such as cerebroside, needed for development of the central nervous system), and promotes the growth of harmless *Lactobacilli* in the intestine thereby making the gut contents relatively acidic. Other carbohydrates are present in much smaller quantities, and include nitrogen-containing carbohydrates such as *bifidus factor* which is much more concentrated in human milk than in cows' milk, and is lost altogether if milk is heated; bifidus factor facilitates the growth of *Lactobacillus bifidus* which develops at the expense of less desirable organisms such as *E. Coli*. The intestinal flora of the breast-fed baby are thus very different from those of the baby fed on cows' milk or its derivatives.

Since cows' milk contains less lactose than human milk, other solutes must be present in higher concentration to ensure isotonicity. The sodium content of human milk is less than a third of that of cows' milk, and thus presents a substantially lower load of solute to be excreted. The high sodium and protein content of cows' milk increases the likelihood of hypernatraemia or uraemia in infants fed on its derivatives; the danger may be exacerbated by the well-intentioned but misguided practice of using over-concentrated feeds to pacify a crying infant who is thought to be hungry, but who is really dehydrated. The consequent sodium retention may lead to water retention which may contribute to rapid weight gain of artificially fed babies. Although human milk has a lower concentration of calcium than cows' milk, the latter is associated with a greater incidence of hypocalcaemia when fed to the neonate. This is due to diminution of calcium absorption from cows' milk: (a) because of the appearance of palmitic acid as a digestion product of bovine triglycerides, leading to the precipitation of calcium palmitate soap in the intestinal lumen, and (b) because of the higher phosphate content in cows' milk which increases the buffering within the intestine, making it more alkaline and therefore more readily colonized by potentially pathogenic bacteria.

Both human and cows' milk contain little iron, but the store of iron in the neonatal liver is large, having risen steeply in the last weeks of pregnancy; the newborn receives a transfusion of placental blood immediately after delivery, and thus an increase in iron stores, immediately after delivery so long as the umbilical cord is not too hastily clamped. The addition of iron to the diet of the infant may saturate the iron-binding protein lactoferrin, making iron available for the metabolism of certain intestinal pathogens.

The vitamin content of human milk varies with the diet of the mother; if maternal diet is satisfactory, human milk provides an adequate source of all vitamins with the possible exception of vitamin D, which may be derived to some extent from ultraviolet irradiation of the baby's skin.

So far as potentially toxic substances in the maternal circulation are concerned, two issues arise: (i) 'Is the substance excreted in any quantity in the milk?' and (ii) ' Does the baby absorb it, and does the substance cause any ill-effects?' The answer to the former question will depend upon the lipid solubility of the substance, and on its tendency to bind to milk rather than to plasma. Ethical considerations make it impossible to produce firm answers to the latter questions, but certain drugs are best avoided during lactation.

Maternal consequences of lactation

Lactation makes greater energy demands on the mother than does pregnancy. The human baby takes twice as long to grow to 3.5 kg before birth as it does to double this weight after birth. Moreover, the provision of nutrients in milk for growth after birth is less efficient than the nutrition of the fetus in the uterus.

The cost of lactation includes not only the nutrients in the milk, but also the energy required for the synthesis of many of the components of milk; the energy efficiency of milk production is about 80–90 per cent. The most important reason for the inefficiency of postnatal nutrition is that much of the energy in milk must be used to maintain the infant's body temperature. In the first 2 months after birth, only 26 per cent of the energy intake is used for growth, and the proportion has fallen to 7 per cent by 4–6 months. Given the daily volumes of milk produced, its energy value and the total energy cost to the mother, it can be calculated that the lactating woman should have 600–800 kcal (2520–3360 kJ) more than her normal daily intake. Some of this will be derived from the fat stored during pregnancy; the 4 kg of fat typically laid down will provide some 36 000 kcal (151 200 kJ) of energy — between a third and a half of the energy needed for the production of breast milk.

The second effect of lactation is the suppression of ovulation. Suckling suppresses release of gonadotrophins thereby causing lack of ovulation and amenorrhoea. The duration of this condition is the greater (a) the more frequent and prolonged the nursing episodes, and (b) the less well-nourished the mother. The consequent contraceptive effect, though it may be unreliable as a birth control method for the individual woman, results in a substantial (about 5–15 month) increase in the mean interval between births in human communities. The effect wanes with time, and ultimately ovulation and menstruation — and thus fertility — return during prolonged breast feeding.

We have referred already to the other major neuroendocrine consequences of lactation — the release of oxytocin and prolactin; suffice it to recall the importance of oxytocin in stimulating myometrial contraction immediately after parturition; this may promote placental separation, reduce uterine haemorrhage, and hasten the return of the uterus to its nonpregnant size and shape.

A third group of effects of lactation on mothers falls into the 'psycho-social' category — the mention of which makes physiologists uneasy. We should not, however, ignore the evidence that a successful lactation may contribute to the quality of the relationship between mother and infant. One reason might be the pleasure that nursing gives to a mother. Nursing, like eating, drinking and coitus, is an action upon which the survival of the species depends: the acts of eating, drinking and coitus are normally gratifying, and such gratification is inextricably linked to the motivation to perform those acts. The motivation to nurse might logically, then, be linked to the gratifying effects to the mother of nursing (and there is evidence to support this view). If the source of this gratification is the infant, it is to be expected that the affection of a mother for her infant would be enhanced by nursing. By this argument, sociobiologists might describe suckling by an infant as a tactic designed to elicit altruistic behaviour from its mother.

Involution of the mammary gland

Involution of mammary tissue can occur (a) if milk removal is suddenly stopped when milk secretion is in full swing; (b) gradually when, having reached a maximum secretion rate, the milk yield declines during the rest of a lactation period; and (c) as a result of advancing age ('senile' or 'post-menopausal' involution). The first form of involution belongs more to pathology than to physiology; it is associated with distension of the breast, alveolar rupture, and a characteristic sequence of histological changes.

Postlactational involution
Gradual involution at the end of a period of lactation is associated with reduction in the infant's appetite for breast milk as other food is introduced. The emergence of the infant's upper incisors (at six to ten months) may cause nursing to become an uncomfortable experience for the mother. The duration of lactation varies; it commonly lasts for three to six months, but may continue for two years or longer. The removal of the infant from the breast (weaning) is associated with a fall of milk secretion and degenerative changes in mammary alveolar cells. Intracellular lysosomal enzymes appear; they eliminate intracellular constituents involved in the secretory process. Phagocytic cells assist in the elimination of necrotic cells and stagnated milk. Connective tissue and fat invade the spaces between the involuted alveoli. The total involutional process lasts two to three months.

Although the suckling stimulus reduces fertility, women can become pregnant whilst lactating; if this happens, nursing is usually stopped by the third month of pregnancy, though it may continue up to the seventh month. The high steroid levels during pregnancy tend to inhibit milk secretion.

Post-menopausal involution
The decline in ovarian steroid secretion at the menopause is associated with a reduction of glandular tissue, an increase in fat deposition, and a relative predominance of connective tissue in the breast. In nonobese postmenopausal women, the breasts shrink to a small mass as a result of regression of glandular tissue. In obese women, glandular tissue is replaced by fat, and there may be no reduction in breast size.

Maternal behaviour

Introduction

Just as the behaviours of courtship and mating are indispensable if ovulation and spermatogenesis are to have their intended outcome, so maternal behaviour is as necessary to the survival of the offspring of most mammals as are lactation and parturition. Indeed without maternal behaviour, lactation will soon fail. There is a growing awareness that in its eagerness to stage-manage the birth and early life of the infant, the medical profession may have lost sight of some simple biological imperatives which govern behaviour.

There are three phases to maternal behaviour: (i) ante-natal behaviour such as nest building (and visiting baby-care shops), (ii) behaviour concerned with the protection, thermoregulation and nutrition of offspring after birth, and (iii) behaviour associated with the gradual independence of offspring.

Ante-natal behaviour

Human behaviour *prior to* parturition is rarely described in the sense that an ethologist would describe animal behaviour, though certain forms of behaviour are either prescribed or proscribed by convention, advertising, or medical advice. Many animals exhibit nest-building, apparently in response to hormonal changes occurring in pregnancy.

Behaviour during parturition

Discussion of human behaviour *during* parturition currently is focussed on the suitability of particular environments (home versus hospital); many animals seek a quiet dark place for parturition. The possible benefits of the supine position for the second stage of labour (i.e. the ease of access by doctors and midwives to the birth canal) must be weighed against the cost of restraining a woman in a fixed posture and increasing her anxiety. Furthermore, venous return from the lower parts of the body may be impeded by the weight of the uterine contents pressing on the vena cava, so leading to a reduced cardiac output and arterial hypotension. In many non-European cultures, women adopt an upright posture, e.g. kneeling or squatting, during delivery.

Postpartum behaviour

Female rats presented postpartum with newborn foster young will respond to them immediately with appropriate behaviour e.g. retrieving if they stray from the nest, crouching over them, and licking. Virgin rats, both male and female, respond similarly only after exposure to pups for about a week. A hormone regimen aimed at mimicking the endocrine changes occurring during pregnancy can cut the latent period down to about 40 hours; the endocrine changes not only prime the rat uterus for parturition and its mammary glands for lactation, but also prime its brain to exhibit maternal behaviour. The brain of the mother immediately after the parturition may therefore be particularly sensitive to stimuli from the neonate which initiate normal patterns of maternal care, and if those stimuli are not presented during the sensitive period, initiation of normal maternal behaviour may not occur. Further evidence for this concept of a postpartum sensitive period is provided by experiments involving separation of newborn sheep and goats from their mothers at various times after birth. If a goat kid is in contact with its mother in the first five minutes after birth, a stable bond will be established between the two, but a kid separated from the mother during the same period will often be rejected.

It used to be considered good practice to separate a mother from her baby for several hours after parturition. It has, however, been claimed that if an hour or more of close physical contact between mothers and their babies is allowed just after delivery, maternal care shows an enduring improvement. Conversely there is a disproportionately high incidence of mothering disturbances, such as child abuse and failure-to-thrive, occurring after mothers have been separated from their newborn infants. Klaus and Kennell must take much credit for highlighting these facts, and for stimulating a reappraisal of the management of the perinatal period in maternity units. A period of close contact between mother and baby after delivery allows *bonding* to take place. *Rooming-in regimes*, with the baby sleeping close to the mother, are encouraged, and a more relaxed attitude is taken to the timing of breast feeding.

The interaction between mother and infant is obviously a two-way process, and disturbance of the relationship can have lasting effects for both. Deprivation of all (though not of some) of the normal components of maternal care can produce lasting behavioural disorders in offspring which will affect their ability to cope with life in general, and, in particular, with the care of their own offspring. A woman's emotional state may be profoundly affected by the experience of parturition and the change in life-style which is the inevitable consequence of caring for a newborn infant (Steele: *Gynaecology, Obstetrics and the Neonate*, Chapter 7).

Further reading

Ciba Foundation Symposium, No. 33 (1975). *Parent-Infant Interaction.* Elsevier/Excerpta Medica/North-Holland, Amsterdam.

Ciba Foundation Symposium, No. 45 (1976). *Breast Feeding and the Mother.* Elsevier/Excerpta Medica/North-Holland, Amsterdam.

Cowie, A.T., Forsyth, I.A. and Hart, I.C. (1980). *Hormonal Control of Lactation.* Springer-Verlag, Berlin.

Gubernick, D.J. and Klopfer, P.H. (eds) (1981). *Parental Care in Mammals.* Plenum, New York.

Jelliffe, D.B. and Jelliffe, E.F.P. (1978). *Human Milk in the Modern World.* Oxford University Press, Oxford.

Klaus, M.H. and Kennell, J.H. (1976). *Maternal-Infant Bonding: the Impact of Early Separation or Loss on Family Development.* C.V. Mosby, St Louis.

Larson, B.L. and Smith, V.R. (eds) (1974 and 1978). *Lactation: A Comprehensive Treatise.* Vols. I, Ii, III, IV. Academic Press, New York.

Lawrence, R.A.(1980). *Breast feeding: a Guide for the Medical Profession.* C.V. Mosby, St Louis.

Mepham, B. (1976). *The Secretion of Milk.* The Institute of Biology's Studies in Biology no. 60. Edward Arnold, London.

Peaker, M. (ed.) (1977). *Comparative Aspects of Lactation.* Academic Press, London.

Vorherr, H. (1975). *The Breast: Morphology, Physiology and Lactation.* Academic Press, New York.

10

The hormones of reproduction

Introduction

This chapter consists of a list of the reproductive hormones and summarizes our knowledge of them. The list does not include a number of hormones, e.g. ACTH, thyroid hormones and corticosteroids which, though not primarily reproductive, affect such functions as fetal maturation, parturition, and lactation.

Each hormone or group of hormones is covered systematically to the extent that information is available. In the case of some poorly understood hormones facts can be provided under only a few headings. Where possible, the following information is provided: other names, most important examples, chemical characteristics, sites of synthesis/release, biosynthesis, mechanism of action, physiological effects, agonists, antagonists, binding, disappearance rate, catabolism and excretion, control of release, causes/effects of deficiency, causes/effects of excess. More detailed information on many of the hormones is given in the first nine Chapters, and can be traced via the Index.

Table 10.1 and Fig. 10.1 provide additional sources for reference. In the former, 'normal' values for plasma concentrations of several major hormones are provided for different stages in reproductive life; this table can usefully be studied in conjunction with Figs 1.9, 3.7, 3.9 and 6.4. Fig. 10.1 can be used either for the study of steroid biosynthesis, or as a source of reference for the chemical formulae of many steroid hormones with reproductive functions.

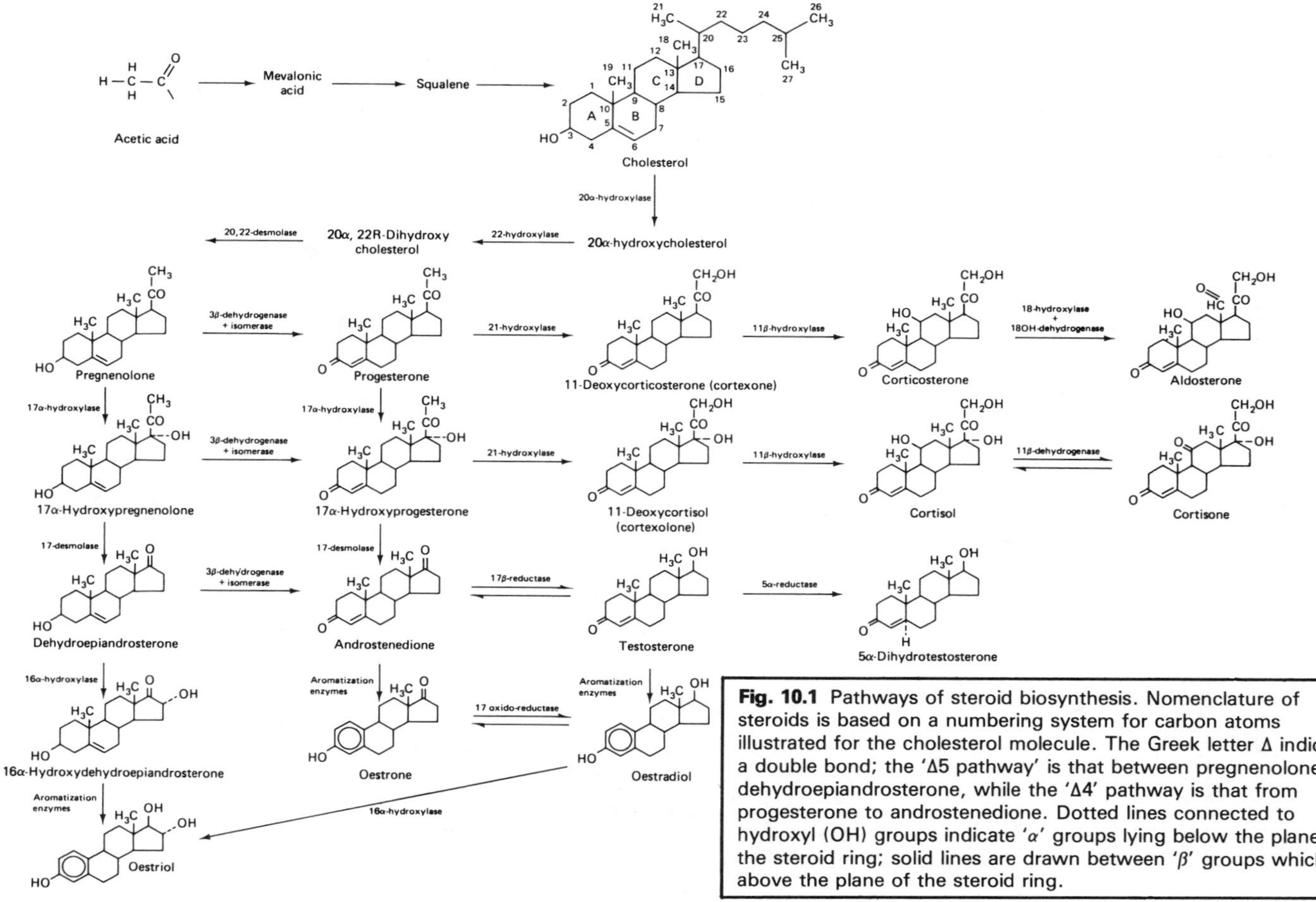

Fig. 10.1 Pathways of steroid biosynthesis. Nomenclature of steroids is based on a numbering system for carbon atoms illustrated for the cholesterol molecule. The Greek letter Δ indicates a double bond; the 'Δ5 pathway' is that between pregnenolone and dehydroepiandrosterone, while the 'Δ4' pathway is that from progesterone to androstenedione. Dotted lines connected to hydroxyl (OH) groups indicate 'α' groups lying below the plane of the steroid ring; solid lines are drawn between 'β' groups which lie above the plane of the steroid ring.

Table 10.1 Typical values and/or ranges of reproductive hormone concentrations in plasma of human males and females at different stages of reproductive life. Note that:
1. In adult males over 65 years, testosterone levels may be 20–40 per cent lower than those in a young man.
2. Values quoted for pituitary hormones refer to UK standard preparations: FSH — NIBSC 69/104; LH — NIBSC 68/40; Prolactin — NIBSC 75/504.

	FSH (U/litre)	LH (U/litre)	Prolactin (mU/litre)	Androstenedione		Testosterone	
				(nmol/l)	(ng/ml)	(nmol/litre)	ng/ml
M 5–9 years, prepuberty, stage P1	<2.0	<1.0	—	—	—	0.3–0.8	0.09–0.23
M 9–11 years, stage P2	<3.0	<1.0	—	—	—	0.8–1.5	0.23–0.43
M 11–14 years, stage P3	<4.0	<3.0	—	—	—	2.5–4.0	0.72–1.15
M 14–16 years, stage P4	<6.0	<8.0	—	—	—	5.0–7.0	1.4–2.0
M Adult	1.5–6	2–12	<150	—	—	10–30	2.9–8.7
F Up to 60 days	9 (2–60)	4 (1.5–9)		—	—	0.5 (<0.8)	0.14 (<0.23)
F 2–12 months	7 (2–60)	3 (1–8)		—	—	0.2 (<0.6)	0.06 (<0.29)
F 1–10 years	4.5 (1–12)	2.3 (1–4)		—	—	0.3 (<0.5)	0.05 (<0.14)
F 10–12 years, stages P1 and P2	6 (3–10)	3 (2–6)		—	—	0.6 (<1.5)	0.17 (<0.43)
F 12–14 years, stage P3	7 (4–11)	5 (1–12)		—	—	1.0 (<2.0)	0.29 (<0.58)
F 14–16 years, stage P4	9 (4–25)	10 (3–50)		—	—	1.0 (<2.5)	0.29 (<0.72)
F Adult, follicular phase of menstrual cycle	2–8	3–10	40–300	4.9	1.4	0.3–2.5	0.09–0.72
F Adult, ovulatory phase of menstrual cycle	6–25	20–70	40–300	6.6	1.9	0.3–2.5	0.09–0.72
F Adult, mid-luteal phase of menstrual cycle	2–6	3–12	40–300	4.9	1.4	0.3–2.5	0.09–0.72
F Adult, climacteric	10–50	10–60	40–300	**Variable**		1.8 (<3.4)	0.52 (<0.98)
F Adult, 1 year post-menopausal	45 (25–70)	55 (35–70)	40–300	1.2 (<3.0)	0.34 (<0.86)	1.8 (<3.4)	0.52 (<0.98)
F Adult, 2–3 years post-menopausal	65 (45–85)	60 (40–80)	40–300	1.2 (<3.0)	0.3 (<0.86)	1.4 (<3.4)	0.40 (<0.98)
F Adult, 5 years post-menopausal	55 (30–80)	55 (35–60)	40–300	1.5 (<3.0)	0.43 (<0.86)	1.0 (<3.4)	0.29 (<0.98)
F Adult, 10 years post-menopausal	45 (30–65)	55 (35–80)	40–300	1.6 (<4.0)	0.46 (<1.5)	1.5 (<3.4)	0.43 (<0.98)
F Adult, 20 years post-menopausal	25 (5–45)	30 (6–50)	40–300	1.5 (<4.0)	0.43 (<1.15)	2.0 (<3.4)	0.58 (<0.98)

3. The stress of anticipation of venepuncture for blood sampling can raise prolactin levels in normal subjects to as high as 700 mU/l. Prolactin has a marked 24-hour rhythmicity, being higher during sleep; values quoted are for daytime.

4. Levels of many hormones, including LH, FSH, prolactin, testosterone and androstenedione can show marked oscillations in concentration with peak levels at two to three times the mean level. Androstenedione and 17-OH-progesterone show a 24-hour rhythmicity being highest between 0700 and 1000 h.

Oestradiol		Oestrone		Progesterone		17-OH Progesterone	
(p mol/litre)	(pg/ml)	(pmol/litre)	(pg/ml)	(nmol/litre)	(ng/ml)	(nmol/litre)	(ng/ml)
—	—	—	—	—	—	—	—
—	—	—	—	—	—	—	—
—	—	—	—	—	—	—	—
—	—	—	—	—	—	—	—
75–295	20–80	4.2	1.2	—	—	—	—
100 (<200)	30 (<55)	—	—	<1	<0.31	3 (1–7)	1.0 (0.2–2.3)
100 (<300)	30 (<82)	—	—	<1	<0.31	2 (1–5)	0.67 (0.3–1.65)
100 (<200)	30 (<55)	—	—	<1	<0.31	1.3 (0.5–3)	0.43 (0.16–1.0)
100 (<300)	30 (<82)	—	—	<2	<0.62	<4	<1.3
200 (<400)	55 (<110)	—	—	<4	<1.26	<7	<2.3
300 (<800)	82 (<220)	—	—	<4–50	<1.62–16	<7	<2.3
40–60	11–16	11	50	<4	<1.26	1.5 (<7)	0.5 (<2.3)
300–1500	82–410	300–660	150–300	<4	<1.26	5.2 (<7)	1.7 (<2.3)
150–1000	40–270	240	110	30–90	9.4–28.3	4.5 (<7)	1.3 (<2.3)
Variable	Variable	Variable	Variable	—	—	—	—
52 (25–145)	14 (7–40)	90 (40–150)	24 (11–41)	—	—	—	—
51 (25–120)	14 (7–33)	65 (37–90)	18 (10–24)	—	—	—	—
50 (25–180)	14 (7–50)	70 (37–155)	19 (10–42)	—	—	—	—
45 (20–90)	12 (5–25)	35 (9–100)	9 (2–27)	—	—	—	—
40 (20–90)	11 (5–25)	40 (25–75)	11 (7–20)	—	—	—	—

Androgens

Most important examples   Testosterone (T; 17β-hydroxyandrost-4-ene-3-one) 5α-dihydrotestosterone (DHT; androstanolone, 17β-hydroxy-5α-androstan-3-one) Androstenedione (Δ4; androst-4-ene-3, 17-dione) Dehydroepiandrosterone (DHA; DHEA)

Chemical characteristics   Natural androgens are steroids with 19 carbon atoms (C19-steroids) with β-methyls at C10 and C13, and, in most cases, oxygen substitutions at C3 and C17.

Sites of synthesis/release   Testosterone from Leydig cells of testis; Δ4 converted to T, especially in liver and adipose tissue. Testis produces smaller amounts of DHEA, Δ4, DHT, and oestrogens. Δ4 also arises from adrenal cortex and ovary. DHEA sulphate secreted by adrenal cortex; arises from fetal zone in adrenal cortex of fetus. DHT produced mainly in cells of certain androgen target organs.

Biosynthesis   Androgens arise from cholesterol along Δ5 and Δ4 pathways; precursors in testis are acetate, cholesterol and lipoproteins. Fetal adrenal uses pregnenolone. Synthesis in testis (mg/day) is:- T, 6; Δ4, 0.5; DHEA, 0.7. Only 10 per cent of total DHT production is from testis; 90 per cent is in target tissues e.g. accessory sex glands, by conversion of T by intracellular 5α-reductase.

Mechanism of action   Androgens enter cells by passive diffusion; only unbound hormone can enter. Before or after intracellular conversion they bind to a specific receptor protein, inducing conformational change to form activated hormone-receptor complex which is translocated to cell nucleus to occupy acceptor sites within nuclear chromatin. Transcription is stimulated providing more ribosomal RNA, more messenger RNA (thus specifying proteins formed during cell response), and more DNA in preparation for cell division. Receptor complex occupies intranuclear acceptor sites for 12–16 hours. In prostate and differentiating external genitalia, T undergoes intracellular conversion by 5α-reductase to DHT which becomes tightly bound to a cytoplasmic androgen receptor which has high affinity for DHT, but low affinity for T. Some androgen target tissues lack 5α-reductase (e.g. vas deferens. muscle, and bone); T exerts a direct effect on these tissues.

In the brain of fetal or neonatal mammals, T produces irreversible changes which cause male behaviour in adulthood and, in rats, non-cyclic gonadotrophin secretion. These effects of T depend on aromatase within cells of hypothalamus which converts T to oestradiol-17β which is bound to oestrogen receptors. T's modulation of gonadotrophin secretion from pituitary may also depend on aromatization.

In the testis, both T and FSH are needed for spermatogenesis. They promote various functions of Sertoli cells including synthesis of androgen binding protein. T is present in high concentrations in vicinity of seminiferous tubules because of close proximity of Leydig cells. T binds to peritubular myoid cells and Sertoli cells, but not to germ cells. Cells of the epididymis are stimulated by androgens to provide an environment permitting sperm maturation.

Physiological effects   Androgenic steroids vary in potency depending on the target organ. DHT regarded as most potent, with T, Δ4, and DHEA having relative potencies of about 50 per cent, 8 per cent and 4 per cent respectively. DHT is very active on prostate, external genitalia and secondary sex hair-bearing skin; T more active on muscle, bone, epididymis, vas deferens, and seminal vesicles. DHT has no androgenic effect on the brain, because it cannot be aromatized to oestradiol. Δ4, often considered a weak androgen, may be converted to T in the liver, for example, to give high tissue concentration in absence of high blood level of T. In the skin, for example, Δ4 is converted to oestrogens. Androgens develop and maintain masculine traits.

In males:

1. Induce and maintain differentiation of somatic tissues e.g. muscle.
2. Induce secondary sex characteristics (deep voice, body hair, penis growth).
3. Induce *and maintain* secondary sex characteristics (development and secretory activity of accessory sex organs).
4. Influence sexual and aggressive behaviour.

5. Support spermatogenesis: precise role uncertain and varies with species. Early differentiation of spermatocytes, final stages of meiotic division, and sperm maturation in epididymis are androgen-dependent (the last also FSH-dependent).
6. Promote protein anabolism, somatic growth, ossification and fusion of epiphyses in bone.
7. Inhibit secretion of gonadotrophins.
8. Stimulate organ-specific protein and enzyme synthesis e.g. in liver, kidney and salivary gland.

In females:
1. Induce body hair at puberty.
2. Influence sexual and aggressive behaviour e.g. libido.

In fetus:
1. DHEA is precursor for placental oestrogen synthesis.
2. T from testis causes male sexual differentiation.

Agonists Some synthetic analogues affect seminal vesicles more powerfully than T (because of less binding to plasma proteins). Fluoride in molecule enhances potency, e.g. fluoxymestrone. Caulesterone used for breast cancer. Danazol a weak androgen, but selectively inhibits pituitary gonadotrophin release. Anabolic steroids e.g. stanozolol, have slight effect on seminal vesicles but maintain skeletal growth.

Antagonists Several anti-androgens are used in treatment hypersexuality, acne, hirsutism, and prostatic cancer:

(a) *Cyproterone* and *cyproterone acetate*: steroids which compete with DHT and block most effects of T and DHT.
(b) *Flutamide*: non-steroid anti-androgen.

Binding Forty per cent of circulating androgens bound to plasma albumin, forty seven per cent to sex-hormone binding globulin (SHBG), 2 per cent free. Sulphated androgens, e.g. DHEA sulphate, bind weakly to albumin only. SHBG levels equal in boys and girls before puberty, but in male adults SHBG is about half that in females. The plasma concentration of T in men is 20 × that in women, but the concentration of *free* T is 40 ×.

Disappearance rate Blood clearance per minute:

T	0.5 litres (women)	0.7 litres (men)
$\Delta 4$	1.3 litres (women)	1.6 litres (men)

Catabolism and excretion Testosterone metabolized in liver to 5α-reduced steroids which are then hydroxylated or conjugated as glucuronides and excreted in urine as 17-ketosteroids. Some conversion to oestrogens.

Control of release Secretion of T from Leydig cells controlled by LH, therefore by all factors controlling LH. Leydig cells bind LH which increases availability of steroid substrate by accelerating cholesterol metabolism. In males, activation of LH secretion causes puberty. A 24-hour rhythmicity of LH secretion present in early puberty, but less obvious in adult men. Testicular androgen production shows seasonal rhythmicity for example, in deer. In male fetus, hCG stimulates production of T by testis.

Adrenal androgen production (notably DHEA and DHEA sulphate) in fetal adrenal cortex accelerates during gestation, but control not understood. After birth, adrenal androgen production in boys and girls increases from the eighth year to the fourteenth year; control of this 'adrenarche' not understood. In post-menopausal women, adrenals secrete DHEA, $\Delta 4$, and T, regulated by ACTH. Ovarian secretion of DHEA and T regulated by gonadotrophins.

Causes/effects of deficiency Deficiency in men causes abnormalities in virility, genitalia and fat distribution. If deficiency prevents puberty, patient has child-like face, lack of beard hair, smooth skin and eunuchoidal proportions arising from delayed epiphyseal fusion. In adults, pallor, skin wrinkling, reduced beard growth, poor musculature and feminine body contours are seen. Defective spermatogenesis and impotence common. Osteoporosis occurs in prolonged deficiency.

Secretion of T may be reduced by a number of drugs including alcohol and heroin. In the fetus, deficiency of 17,20 desmolase (required for androgen synthesis) causes low androgen output; sexual differentiation of male fetus fails. Deficiency of 5α-reductase causes defective conversion of T to DHT; affected male infants have poorly developed male external genitalia. At puberty, external genitalia suddenly exposed to higher levels of T and grow normal size — the so-called 'penis at twelve' syndrome, but infertility remains.

Deficiency of *effects* of androgens may arise from defective development of androgen receptors in 'testicular feminization' (Fig. 1.2c): patients have XY-chromosome constitution, abdominal testes secreting greater than normal amounts of T and oestradiol-17β, and female body form; often married, with normal gender identity, behaviour, external genitalia, and well-developed breasts. Their tissues fail to respond to androgens although secreted and present in blood.

Causes/effects of excess   In foetus, excess corticosteroid production results in excess androgen which masculinizes female foetuses (Fig. 1.2d). Precocious puberty in males often results from excess adrenal androgen production. In adult females, over-production of androgens by adrenal cortex or ovary causes virilization (Steele: *Gynaecology, Obstetrics and the Neonate*, Chapter 18).

Follicle stimulating hormone (FSH)

Chemical characteristics   Glycoprotein (carbohydrate 27 per cent; sialic acid 5 per cent); mol. wt approx. 33 000. Two dissimilar subunits:

αsubunit: 89 AAs, 2 carbohydrate chains (structure identical to α subunit of hCG, LH, and TSH).
βsubunit: 115 AAs, 2 carbohydrate chains (confers specificity).

Site of synthesis/release   Anterior pituitary basophilic gonadotrophs (comprise 5 per cent of anterior pituitary cells).

Biosynthesis   By ribosomal synthesis of peptide chains, with addition of carbohydrate residues in rough endoplasmic reticulum. Addition of terminal sugar residues in Golgi apparatus.

Mechanism of action   Binds to target cells, activates adenylate cyclase, causing increase in intracellular cAMP and thus accelerated end-product synthesis (including, in granulosa cells, LH receptors).

Physiological effects   Receptors in female only in granulosa cells of follicle (where they develop during earliest stage of follicular development); on male only in Sertoli cells of seminiferous tubule.

FSH in female stimulates follicular development from antral to pre-ovulatory stage. Pure FSH will not promote steroid secretion from developing follicles. Follicle stimulating hormone initiates fluid movement within ovarian follicles and into seminiferous tubules. Stimulates protein synthesis and increases mitotic activity in growing follicles; this effect potentiated by oestrogens. Follicle stimulating hormone acts on follicle to promote growth and maturation, and increases number of LH binding sites on granulosa cells. Follicle stimulating hormone *and* LH cause resumption of meioses, induction of ovulation, increase of cAMP within granulosa cells, and progesterone accumulation. Follicle stimulating hormone stimulates production of plasminogen activator from granulosa cells as ovulation approaches, so contributing to breakdown of follicle wall which precedes ovum release. Follicle stimulating hormone stimulates aromatization in granulosa cells which converts androgens to oestrogens.

In male, FSH stimulates growth of seminiferous tubules. Site of action is Sertoli cells where, with testosterone, FSH stimulates production of androgen-binding protein (ABP) and other functions. Sertoli cells then influence germ cells. This effect most important at initiation of spermatogenesis; sperm production in adults apparently not controlled by FSH.

Disappearance rate   Plasma half-life about 3 hours.

Catabolism and excretion   Little known, but liver and kidney important.

Control of release   Both FSH and LH are released in response to single hypothalamic hormone (GnRH) (q.v.). Sensitivity of pituitary to GnRH influenced by steroid hormones; effects may differ for FSH and LH, and levels of the two hormones may be dissociated. Secretion of FSH rises when ovarian follicle activity absent (e.g. after the menopause); follicle may produce an 'inhibin' like that from testis to control FSH secretion. The release of FSH is pulsatile, but pulses smaller than those of LH. Changes in secretion of ovarian steroids and/or hypothalamic GnRH, which cause the mid-cycle surge of LH, cause a similar, if less marked, surge in FSH secretion.

Causes/effects of deficiency Isolated FSH deficiency is rare. More often FSH *and* LH are affected by deficient GnRH production (as in Kallman's syndrome). In polycystic ovary syndrome, and in presence of oestrogen-secreting tumours, FSH secretion is low. The levels of FSH are reduced in anorexia nervosa.

Deficiency of gonadotrophins: in women during reproductive life causes amenorrhoea (Steele: *Gynaecology, Obstetrics and the Neonate*, Chapter 16) and loss of pubic hair; in men, impotence and testicular atrophy; in children of both sexes, puberty delayed or absent.

Causes/effects of excess Excess endogenous release or exogenous administration of FSH and/or LH (e.g. during treatment for infertility) may cause multiple ovulations and ovarian cysts. At climacteric, high levels of FSH may cause vasomotor symptoms, e.g. hot flushes. High FSH found in patients with amenorrhoea secondary to ovarian failure, e.g. after menopause (Steele: *Gynaecology, Obstetrics and the Neonate*, Chapter 16).

Gonadotrophin-releasing hormone (GnRH)

Other names Luteorelin, gonadorelin, luteinizing hormone releasing hormone or factor (LHRH or LRF).

Chemical characteristics Decapeptide; mol. wt 1182.33 PyroGlu-His-Trp-Ser-Tyr-Gly-Leu-Arg-Pro-Gly-NH$_2$

Sites of synthesis/release Found in neuron cell bodies in suprachiasmatic/ preoptic region and medial basal hypothalamus, including median eminence. Also in organum vasculosum of the lamina terminalis (OVLT) and pineal. Release by axon terminals into primary portal capillaries in median eminence; also may be transported to those capillaries by tanycyte ependymal cells from third ventricular CSF.

Biosynthesis Larger prohormone synthesized on ribosomes, then broken down to active hormones by peptidases.

Mechanism of action Attachment to membrane receptor. Receptor availability may be regulated by gonadal steroids. Cyclic AMP probably acts as intracellular mediator which activates a protein kinase; this changes membrane permeability increasing influx of Ca^{2+}. GnRH probably induces rapid release of readily releasable pool of gonadotrophin by exocytosis, followed by release of stored or newly synthesized hormones; i.e. overall effect on synthesis and release of FSH and LH.

Physiological effects The pituitary gland is stimulated by GnRH to induce, in women, ovulation of suitably primed Graafian follicle and, in men, stimulation of testicular function. This achieved by stimulating FSH and LH release. Target cell is gonadotroph of anterior pituitary gland (about 5 per cent of the cell population) which secretes both FSH and LH. GnRH increases gonadotroph sensitivity to GnRH—a 'self-priming effect'. May also be a CNS neurotransmitter.

Agonists Amino acid substitutions can increase potency 30–100 times, and confer greater resistance to enzymic attack. Theophylline and exogenous cAMP can mimic GnRH effects.

Antagonists Produced by modifying positions His^2, Trp^3, and Gly^6 in the GnRH molecule, but potency insufficient for clinical application in contraception. Steroid contraceptives (or endogenous steroids) may decrease pituitary responsiveness to GnRH.

Disappearance rate Half-life 4–5 minutes.

Catabolism and excretion Mainly inactivated in tissues, and only slowly in the plasma. GnRH metabolized before excretion, several peptides derived from it identified in urine.

Control of release Multifactorial and complex; see Chapters 2,3 and 4. In summary:

1. Circulating gonadal steroids (or synthetic analogues) stimulate or inhibit ovulation via, in part, effect on GnRH release.

2. Suckling inhibits.

3. Coitus stimulates — in rabbit and cat; possibly in human.

4. Severe stress normally inhibits.

5. Light rhythms (seasonal and 24-hour) may affect release in sheep and rat, and probably in man. Seasonal effects probably mediated by pineal, via production of indoles and peptides — especially melatonin which inhibit GnRH secretion. Pineal stimulated by decrease in day-length. Twenty-four hour rhythmicity probably involves the suprachiasmatic nucleus of the hypothalamus.

6. Olfactory stimuli affect GnRH release.

7. Psychic factors may stimulate e.g. in men, anticipation of female company.

8. All systems involved in onset of puberty (e.g. the amygdaloid nuclei, the pineal body, body weight, light levels).

9. Nutrition affects ovulation, probably by affecting GnRH release.

10. Neurotransmitters e.g. noradrenaline and dopamine affect GnRH release. Prostaglandins and γ-aminobutyric acid may stimulate secretion.

Causes/effects of deficiency   Ovulation failure, thus infertility, could arise from lack of GnRH (Steele: *Gynaecology, Obstetrics and the Neonate,* Chapter 15). The release of GnRH is deficient in women with olfactogenital (Kallman's) syndrome, and may be modified in anorexia nervosa.

Human chorionic gonadotrophin (hCG)

Chemical characteristics   Mol. wt. approx. 36 700

Glycoprotein (carbohydrates 30 per cent; sialic acid 8.5 per cent. Two dissimilar sub-units:

α sub-unit: 89 AAs, 2 carbohydrate chains (structure identical to sub-unit of FSH, LH, and TSH)
β sub-unit: 147 AAs (confers specificity; is similar to LH for the first 120 AAs, but tail of 30 unique AAs at N terminal).

Site of synthesis/release   Syncytiotrophoblast and cytotrophoblast cells of placenta (and tumours of trophoblast origin e.g. choriocarcinoma).

Biosynthesis   Individual sub-units of the molecule may be secreted, and placenta secretes large quantities of the α sub-units. Synthesis of whole molecule by normal methods for intracellular protein synthesis on ribosomes. Does not involve secretory granules or Golgi apparatus since specific antisera or lectins do not react with these structures.'

Mechanism of action   Same as LH (q.v.).

Physiological effects   Acts on LH receptors to mimic some, but not all, LH actions; also has weak FSH activity. Effects include:-

1. Maintenance of corpus luteum of pregnancy. Supplements low pituitary LH levels during luteal phase, and overcomes possible luteolytic effects of endogenous ovarian production of oestrogens and protaglandins.

2. Stimulation of fetal testis (important in providing androgens for early sexual differentiation) and of fetal zone of the fetal adrenal gland. These effects made possible by entry of hCG into fetal circulation, especially during weeks 9–3 of pregnancy.

3. Weak ovarian follicle stimulation — but whereas granulosa cells in large follicles bind both FSH and hCG, those in smaller follicles bind only FSH. hCG will include ovulation in follicles primed with FSH.

4. Inhibition of *in vitro* lymphocyte-stimulating effect of phytohaemagglutinin — evidence, perhaps, of some immunosuppressive action. Can also prolong survival of skin grafts in mice.

5. Possible maternal adrenotrophic effects.

6. Stimulates aromatization of androgens to oestrogens by placenta — possible role in regulating placental oestrogen production.

7. Stimulates placental conversion of cholesterol to pregnenolone and progesterone.

8. Possibly inhibits gonadotrophin secretion by maternal pituitary gland in early pregnancy.

Disappearance rate   Disappears from circulation with two-component time course — one with half-life of 20–37 h, the other 5–16 h.

Catabolism and excretion   Excreted in urine; concentration in urine follows pattern similar to that in plasma: urine assays used in pregnancy tests.

Control of release Little known

Causes/effects of excess High levels in multiple pregnancies.

Human placental lactogen (hPL)

Other names Human chorionic somatomammotrophin (hCS)

Chemical characteristics Single chain polypeptide; 191 AAs; mol. wt 22 308 Sequence known; like growth hormone and prolactin.

Site of synthesis/release Syncytiotrophoblast of placenta; production rate up to 1 g/day. Released mainly into maternal circulation, but found in large amounts in amniotic fluid.

Biosynthesis Syncytiotrophoblast has well-developed endoplasmic reticulum, many ribosomes and well-developed Golgi apparatus — suggesting normal ribosomal synthesis of peptide chains, with addition of carbohydrate residues in endoplasmic reticulum and Golgi apparatus.

Mechanism of action/physiological effects hPL cannot readily enter the fetal circulation, so its actions are confined to the mother:

1. Weak (cf. prolactin) stimulation of mammary growth.

2. Growth hormone-like effects on e.g. adipose tissue to promote lipolysis, causing rise in plasma triglycerides and FFAs. Somatotrophic potency of hPL about 0.1–3 per cent of that of growth hormone. hPL inhibits insulin's actions on glucose utilization, but enehances amino acid incorporation. Net effect to conserve glucose, making more available to fetus.

3. Possibly suppression of immunological rejection of fetus by mother. hPL inhibits phytohaemagglutinin-induced lymphocyte transformation, which indicates role in suppression of cell-mediated immune reactions.

4. Probable role, with hCG, in maintenance of corpus luteum of pregnancy.

5. May decrease permeability of amniotic membrane to water, possibly by inhibiting sodium transport.

Agonists Some actions mimicked by prolactin and growth hormone

Disappearance rate Disappearance curves multiexponential; half-life of major component about 12 minutes.

Catabolism and excretion Very little hPL in maternal urine.

Control of release Steady rise in maternal concentration correlated with placental size. Prolonged fasting in mid-pregnancy raises hPL levels.

Causes/effects of deficiency Low hPL levels may indicate defective placental function; low levels sometimes found with fetal distress, threatened abortion, and 'high-risk' pregnancies.

Causes/effects of excess High levels in twin pregnancy, and in non-diabetic pregnancies with excessively large babies. Ectopic production of hPL from tumour tissue possible in males and females.

Inhibin

Other names X-hormone; androhormone; folliculostatin (referring to inhibin from the ovarian follicle)

Chemical characteristics Protein; mol. wt uncertain (1200-160 000). Neither purified, nor structurally characterized.

Sites of synthesis/release Obtained from ovarian or testicular extracts, and from follicular fluid, rete testis fluid, testicular lymph, and semen. Made by Sertoli cells, and probably by granulosa cells of ovarian follicle.

Mechanism of action/physiological effects Acts on the pituitary gland to inhibit FSH secretion. Inhibin and steroids may act synergistically, or one may provide coarse control and the other fine tuning. A tubular factor, possibly inhibin, may also affect the sensitivity of Leydig cells to LH. Existence in primates not accepted by all.

Control of release   In males, secretion of inhibin by Sertoli cells influenced by the presence of germ cells. In females, number of active follicles, and in particular number of granulosa cells, is important. Secretion of inhibin into ovarian venous blood may depend on stage of cycle.

Causes/effects of deficiency   Secretion falls when germinal cells are depleted i.e. in postmenopausal women and aspermatogenic men, evidenced by selective rises in FSH levels.

Luteinizing hormone

Other names   LH; Interstitial cell stimulating hormone (ICSH)

Chemical characteristics   Mol.wt approx. 29 000. Glycoprotein (carbohydrate 16.4 per cent; sialic acid 1.4 per cent). Two dissimilar subunits:

subunit: 89 AAs, 2 carbohydrate chains (identical to subunit of FSH, hCG and TSH)

subunit: 115 AAs, 1 carbohydrate chain (confers specificity).

Site of synthesis/release   Anterior pituitary basophilic gonadotrophs (comprise 5% of anterior pituitary cells).

Biosynthesis   Luteinizing hormone probably formed from prohormone, cleavage of which would result in two subunits and one subunit.

Mechanism of action   Leydig cells of testis possess LH-specific surface receptors. Thecal cells of ovarian follicles develop LH receptors towards end or first phase of development; LH acts on them to stimulate steroidogenesis, especially synthesis of androgens. Oestrogens and FSH cause development of LH-binding sites on follicular granulosa cells during antral phase; during preovulatory phase, surge of LH stimulates both thecal and granulosa cells, initially stimulating, but then stopping, steroidogenic activity of thecal cells; aromatization in granulosa cells also switched off, and their synthesis of progesterone stimulated.

Physiological effects   In male, main function is to stimulate Leydig (interstitial) cells of the testis to produce T, so exerting many androgenic effects. One result is normal progress of spermatogenesis, ensured by high concentration of T near seminiferous tubules.

In female LH stimulates steroid synthesis by all cell types of ovary, but depends on development of LH receptors by cells. Basal levels of LH probably needed for ovarian steroid synthesis, and adequate tonic levels of LH and FSH needed to prevent preantral follicles from becoming atretic. Primary action of LH is stimulation of conversion of cholesterol to pregnenolone; ovary depleted of cholesterol (and ascorbic acid) after LH administration. Other effects include large increase in ovarian blood flow, and stimulation of meiotic and cytoplasmic maturation of oocyte (but LH does not bind directly to oocyte). Possibly neutralizes, or decreases production of, a meiosis-inhibiting factor which may act by reducing cAMP levels in oocyte; might activate, or increase production of, an oocyte maturation factor.

Agonists   Granulosa cells from pre-ovulatory follicles contain receptors for both FSH and LH; FSH can mimic the activity of LH on follicles i.e. progesterone accumulation, resumption of meiosis, and induction of ovulation. hCG mimics many LH effects. Human menopausal gonadotrophin (hMG), extracted from urine of post-menopausal women, contains both FSH and LH. *Clomiphene*, which binds to pituitary oestrogen receptors, stimulates endogenous LH release.

Antagonists   Contraceptive steroids suppress endogenous LH release.

Disappearance rate   Half-life 30 minutes.

Catabolism and excretion   Excreted in urine

Control of release   Rapid LH release follows action of GnRH on anterior pituitary cells. Sensitivity of pituitary cells to GnRH altered by oestrogens and progesterone. High levels of oestrogens *stimulate* LH release. Progesterone in high levels inhibits LH release. Pituitary sensitivity to GnRH increases with exposure ('self-priming' effect). LH may exert negative feedback effect on its own secretion via inhibition of hypothalamic GnRH secretion. The many stimuli affecting GnRH secretion from hypothalamus also influence LH secretion from anterior pituitary.

In rat, ovulatory surge of LH release blocked if the connections between median eminence and preoptic area and adjacent hypothalamic area (PO-AHA) are cut, but tonic LH secretion continues. Therefore PO-AHA responsible for ovulatory surge, but medial basal hypothalamus controls tonic LH levels. In rhesus monkey, both ovulatory and oestrogen-induced LH surges remain if PO-AHA lesioned. Therefore both surge and tonic secretion of LH originate from medial basal hypothalamus or from pituitary gland. Timing of LH surge synchronized to particular phase of the 24-hour day in rat, and maybe also in women.

Causes/effects of deficiency LH (and FSH) deficiency in males seen in Kallmann's syndrome — an inherited condition associated with anosmia. Familial gonadotrophin deficiency described in males and females. LH deficiency in women normally causes amenorrhoea (Steele: *Gynaecology, Obstetrics and the Neonate*, Chapter 16), resulting from ovarian failure, and loss of pubic hair. Women with severe weight loss (resulting from anorexia) release little or no LH even after pituitary stimulation with GnRH. Impotence and testicular atrophy seen in males with LH deficiency. In children of both sexes, puberty absent or delayed.

Causes/effects of excess In polycystic ovary syndrome (Steele: *Gynaecology, Obstetrics and the Neonate*, Chapter 16) LH levels often raised; these patients show exaggerated release of LH after GnRH administration. Over-production of gonadotrophins resulting from hypothalamic-pituitary lesions causes precocious puberty.

Müllerian inhibiting hormone

Other names Müllerian duct inhibiting factor, anti-Müllerian hormone, Müllerian regression factor.

Chemical characteristics Large protein; mol.wt 200 000–230 000

Site of synthesis Sertoli cells of fetal testis

Physiological effects Regression of Müllerian ducts i.e. embryonic female reproductive tract. Unilateral effect if one fetal testis removed.

Control of release Müllerian duct regression first observed at 8 weeks

in male fetuses; complete by the 10th week. Release of hormone independent of pituitary and placental hormones, and continues after birth.

Causes/effects of deficiency A genetic male with androgen-secreting testes may have either defective production of Müllerian inhibiting hormone, or inability of Müllerian duct derivatives to respond to it; result is male with testes, differentiated Wolffian ducts, and normal external genitalia — but also uterus and Fallopian tubes.

Causes/effects of excess Absence of uterus and Fallopian tubes in otherwise normal females may result from production of hormone by nontesticular tissue.

Oestrogens

Most important examples Oestradiol-17β (1,3,5(10)-oestratriene-3-17β-diol; E_2; estradiol).
Oestriol (1,3,5(10)-oestratriene-3,16α,17β-triol; E_3; estriol).
Oestrone (3-hydroxy-1,3,5(10)-oestratriene-17-one;E_1; estrone).

Chemical characteristics Steroids with 18 carbon atoms (C-18 steroids). Aromatic A-ring with a phenolic group in position 3.

Sites of synthesis/release In non-pregnant woman E_2 mainly from ovarian follicle, by cooperation of theca interna and granulosa cells. Thecal cells synthesize androgens but only limited amount of oestrogens. Androgens are precursors for aromatization to oestrogens in granulosa cells. Oestrogens produced by corpus luteum in women — probably by thecal cells incorporated after collapse of follicle.

Some oestrogens which stimulate endometrium at implantation may come from conceptus. In pregnant women placenta produces mainly E_3, but some E_2 and E_1. Fetal liver may synthesize another oestrogen, oestetrol, from placental E_2. E_3 and E_1 produced by E_2 metabolism in liver of nonpregnant women.

In men and post-menopausal women, circulating oestrogens (especially E_1) arise from peripheral conversion of androgens e.g. Δ 4 and T. In men some E_1 comes from adrenal cortex. Thus adrenal cortical hormones, directly and via peripheral conversion, have oestrogenic effects.

Biosynthesis Requires provision of C19 precursors (androgens) to be aromatized to oestrogens. Precursors for ovarian oestrogen production are T and $\Delta 4$ arising from acetate or cholesterol in ovarian thecal and interstitial cells. Main precursor for placental oestrogen synthesis is 16-hydroxydihydroepiandrosterone sulphate from fetal adrenal and fetal liver (where hydroxylation occurs); it is hydrolysed by sulphatase, converted to $\Delta 4$-3-ketone, then aromatized to E_3. Some DHEAS passes to placenta without hydroxylation; it is precursor for E_1 and E_2. Placenta also uses $\Delta 4$ for E_1 synthesis. Ten per cent of oestrogen synthesis in placenta uses DHEAS from maternal adrenal cortex.

Mechanism of action Diffuse into target cells, bind to cytoplasmic high-affinity receptor protein, and convert it to active form. Activated oestrogen-receptor complex translocated to nucleus, binds to chromatin, and enhances production and utilization of messenger and preribosomal RNAs needed for synthesis of constituent, enzymic and secretory proteins, including receptor protein.

Physiological effects Ratio of potency of E_2, E_1 and E_3 roughly 100 : 10 : 1 Oestrogens typically:

1. Stimulate growth and development of female reproductive organs, especially the uterus, vagina and mammary glands.

2. Promote uterine blood supply, protein synthesis, cell division, growth, and myometrial excitability and contractility. Proliferation and secretion of watery fluid by endometrium.

3. Act on lumen of oviduct promoting growth and secretory activity of ciliated epithelial cells. Increase activity of oviductal muscle. Large doses disturb gamete and embryo transport in oviduct causing premature expulsion of the embryo into uterus. If pregnancies occur after large doses of oestrogens, high percentage may occur ectopically owing to 'tube-locking' of embryo caused by oviductal muscle spasm.

4. Cause cervix to become more vascular and oedematous and enhance secretory activity of cervical epithelium. Mucus from oestrogen-treated cervix is profuse and thin, and can be stretched to considerable lengths before threads snap — a high 'Spinnbarkeit' — and forms a 'ferning' pattern as it dries on microscope slide. These changes enhance penetrability of cervix.

5. Induce increased mitotic activity in surface columnar epithelium of vagina, and tendency to keratinize. Hence possible, especially in rodents, to determine stage of ovarian cycle by examination of cell types in smears from vaginal epithelium. Vaginal fluids altered by oestrogens, thus changing metabolic substrates for vaginal bacterial flora; hence altered production of volatile aliphatic acids, so odours may change, causing alterations in sexual attractiveness of female.

6. With progesterone secreted by corpus luteum, may stimulate the endometrium in early pregnancy to release embryotrophic factors needed for activation of conceptus before implantation. Some oestrogens acting in this way may come from embryo.

7. Acting on the uterus towards the end of pregnancy:

(a) Increase actin and myosin synthesis, and storage of energy-rich phosphate, in myometrial cells.

(b) Increase lysosomal instability, thereby increasing activity of phospholipase A, and providing more precursor for, and stimulating synthesis and release of, prostaglandins.

(c) Increase development of myometrial oxytocin and α-adrenaline receptors.

(d) Increase blood flow.

(e) Increase membrane ion transport, thereby increasing membrane potential of myometrial cells from low levels seen in absence of oestrogens.

(f) Possibly increase the development of 'nexuses' (tight junctions) between neighbouring myometrial cells, thereby promoting propagation of excitation.

8. Exert complex action on hypothalamus and anterior pituitary regulating gonadotrophin secretion. Low (but not subnormal) levels of E_2 inhibit gonadotrophin secretion; this 'negative feedback' effect is rapid in onset, detectable within one hour and maximal by 4–6 hours. High E_2 levels *stimulate* gonadotrophin release after a delay. This effect sometimes called 'positive feedback', but delay in gonadotrophin release means

that, in normal ovarian cycle, once the surge in gonadotrophin levels has begun, the follicle has passed the developmental stage when it responds to rising gonadotrophin levels by increasing oestrogen output. Thus components needed to complete 'positive feedback' loop not present; perhaps better to describe this action of oestrogens as 'stimulatory'.

9. Cause somatic effects associated with female secondary sexual characteristics e.g. pelvic enlargement, generalized fat distribution, formation of bone matrix by osteoblasts and epiphyseal closure in growing bones. Depress appetite and exert mild anabolic effect, influence vascular permeability, and cause tissue oedema (particularly in the sexual skin of monkeys).

10. Reduce capillary fragility, blood cholesterol level, and incidence of coronary thrombosis. May increase ability of cardiovascular system to withstand high blood pressures, though maintained elevated levels of oestrogens e.g. during pregnancy or contraceptive therapy, may cause hypertension and increase readiness of blood to clot.

11. Increase activity of renin-angiotensin system.

12. During pregnancy induce widespread changes in maternal metabolism, protein synthesis, and thyroid and adrenal functions. Increase synthesis of steroid-binding protein by maternal liver; so a rise in blood cortisol levels.

13. In mammary gland, promote growth of duct system. With progesterone, they induce lobular-alveolar proliferation.

14. In ovary, stimulate development of LH- and oestrogen-receptors in granulosa cells, increase their mitotic activity, and increase ovarian weight. Exert luteolytic effect on corpus luteum.

15. On many reproductive tissues, induce synthesis of progesterone receptors; hence need for 'priming' of tissues by oestrogens before they can respond to progesterone.

16. Act on brain to influence sexual behaviour. E_2 selectively concentrated in certain areas, e.g. medial preoptic area, arcuate nucleus, ventromedial nucleus, and medial and cortical amygdaloid nuclei. Oestrogens alter activity of neurons in hypothalamus and other brain areas. Oddly enough, E_2 *masculinizes* the fetal brain in many mammals, being produced within the brain by aromatase enzymes from T derived from the fetal testes.

17. Enhance release of prolactin from anterior pituitary, and oxytocin from posterior pituitary. This effect occurs at end of pregnancy as result of rise in oestrogen : progesterone ratio.

Agonists
1. Synthetic derivatives of stilbenes e.g. *diethylstilboestrol* and *hexoestrol*.
2. Modifications of E_2 molecule to enhance stability e.g. *ethinyloestradiol* and *mestranol* used in oral contraceptives (Steele: *Gynaecology, Obstetrics and the Neonate*, Chapter 15).
3. Oestrogenic lactones e.g. *coumestrol* in certain plants.

Antagonists   Conventionally anti-oestrogens do not include 'physiological' antagonists, e.g. androgens and progestagens, but are specific blockers of oestrogens at effector sites. Therapeutic indications for the use of oestrogen antagonists include infertility and hormone-dependent tumours, and they may be used as anti-fertility drugs. Many anti-oestrogens are partial agonists.

One group of anti-oestrogens, the polycyclic phenols, display persistent binding to oestrogen receptors; they include *clomiphene, tamoxifen, ethamoxytriphetol (MER-25)*, and *nafoxidene*. The other group are 'impeded oestrogens', which interact with receptor but dissociate from it too rapidly to exert a strong oestrogenic effect. If present in very high *local* concentrations e.g. in vagina, they block or 'impede' access of E_2 to site of action; they are ineffective systemically; they include steroidal oestrogens such as E_3, and derivatives of diethylstilboestrol such as *dimethylstilboestrol*.

Binding E_1 and E_3 mainly to albumin only; E_2 about equally to albumin and sex-hormone binding globulin, leaving about 1 per cent free.

Disappearance rate   Blood clearance per min: E_2, 1 litre; E_1, 1.5 litres.

Catabolism and excretion E_2 converted to E_1, which undergoes hydroxylation at various carbons including C16 (to give E_3), and reduction of C17 ketone — both followed by conjugation. About 10 per cent excreted as urinary oestrogen glucuronates. Most E_3 excreted as sulphates, glucuronates or sulphoglucuronates.

Control of release   In ovary, two cell types mainly concerned in biosynthesis — theca and granulosa — controlled by LH and FSH respectively, and optimal biosynthesis needs both hormones. All factors (age, neural, environmental, steroid feedback, etc.) influencing secretion of gonadotrophins will influence oestrogen synthesis.

In human placenta, oestrogen synthesis limited by rate at which the fetus provides precursors; control of that process poorly understood. In sheep placenta, E_2 synthesis rises sharply at end of gestation following induction of synthetic enzymes — 17 α-hydroxylase, C_{17-20} lyase and, possibly, aromatases — by cortisol from fetal adrenal cortex.

Causes/effects of deficiency (Steele: *Gynaecology, Obstetrics and the Neonate*, Chapter 21).   Reduced oestrogen levels after menopause cause changes in skin, lack of vaginal secretion, and osteoporosis (Steele: *Gynaecology, Obstetrics and the Neonate*, Chapter 14).

Since E_3 derived from placenta by cooperative biosynthetic activity with fetus, maternal plasma levels of E_3 used as indicator of fetal wellbeing. Low maternal oestrogens during pregnancy may be caused by congenital adrenal hypoplasia of fetus, major fetal CNS malformation, Down's syndrome fetus, and associated with severe anaemia. Low maternal oestrogens may be seen with normal fetal development in cases of placental sulphatase deficiency. *Ampicillin* and glucocorticoids may lower maternal oestrogen levels during pregnancy.

Causes/effects of excess   Synthetic oestrogens (normally administered with progestagens) may interfere with normal tubular transport of fertilized eggs (acting as post-coital contraceptives — 'morning after' pills), or suppress lactation. Also widely used in conventional oral contraceptives (Steele: *Gynaecology, Obstetrics and the Neonate*, Chapter 15). Undesirable side effects may include susceptibility to neoplastic growth (particularly endometrial hyperplasia which may lead to carcinoma), and deep vein thrombosis.

Oxytocin

Chemical characteristics   Octapeptide;
mol. wt 1007.23

$$(NH2)\ Gly–Leu–Pro–Cys — S — S — Cys$$
$$Asp(NH_2)–Glu(NH_2)–Ile–Tyr$$

Site of synthesis/release   Synthesis in cell bodies of paraventricular and supraoptic nuclei of hypothalamus. Hormone then transported within membrane-bound granules combined with specific binding protein or *neurophysin*; oxytocin bound to neurophysin I or 'oestrogen-stimulated neurophysin'. Oxytocin widely distributed in CNS as neurotransmitter, e.g. in cerebellum. Oxytocin released in neurohypophysis by calcium-dependent stimulus-secretion coupling when action potentials reach nerve terminals. Oxytocin released from fetal pituitary during parturition.

Biosynthesis   Synthesized from constituent amino acids, bound to protein, and incorporated into secretory granules.

Mechanism of action   On myometrium: increases sodium permeability of cells causing depolarization; lowers threshold amount of depolarization needed to initiate action potential; increases calcium influx so promoting more powerful contraction; increases release of prostaglandins, esp. $PGF_{2\alpha}$. Sensitivity of myometrium to oxytocin is greatly altered by oestrogens and progesterone.

Similar actions on myoepithelial cells of mammary gland, but less sensitive to variations in steroid levels.

Physiological effects   Contraction of myoepithelial cells in mammary gland (hence milk ejection), and of myometrium (the word 'oxytocin' derived from Greek meaning 'quick birth'). Weak antidiuretic action (about 1 per cent that of ADH), and weak effect of peripheral vascular tone. No known function in male.

Agonists   Some prostaglandins (e.g. E_2 and $F_{2\alpha}$) oxytocic at any stage of pregnancy; may be used for induction of abortions. Oral PGE_2 has been used for induction of labour. Two ergot derivatives, *ergonovine (ergometrine)* and *methylergonovine* are potent oxytocics used to prevent postpartum haemorrhage. *Sparteine* a potent oxytocic.

Antagonists   Labour may be suppressed by inhibiting *release* of oxytocin by intravenous infusion of ethanol. Several 'tocolytic' drugs may antagonize effects of oxytocin by relaxing myometrium. β_2-sympathomimetic drugs (e.g. *ritodrine*) and direct smooth muscle relaxants (e.g. *diazoxide*) used to limited extent. In mammary myoepithelium, catecholamines (e.g. noradrenaline) may inhibit effect of oxytocin.

Binding Not clear whether oxytocin bound to plasma protein.

Disappearance rate Half-life in normal men and nonpregnant women is 3–6 minutes.

Catabolism and excretion Rapidly destroyed by plasma oxytocinase.

Control of release (Fig. 9.3) Distension of the vagina during parturition causes reflex release; plasma levels rise in second stage of labour. Suckling causes release; afferent pathway being via sensory nerves from nipple and surrounding skin. Release inhibited by emotional stress, and by high blood levels of alcohol. Sounds, sights, and thoughts associated with nursing may cause release.

Causes/effects of deficiency Lactation failure follows failure of milk ejection which may result if oxytocin release is inhibited by e.g. emotional stress. Failure of release may prolong parturition.

Causes/effects of excess Pharmacological doses have transient relaxing effect on vascular smooth muscle, and so lower blood pressure. Premature or excess dosage with oxytocin for induction or acceleration of labour can contribute to fetal asphyxia, premature delivery or uterine rupture (Steele: *Gynaecology, Obstetrics and the Neonate*, Chapter 2).

Progestagens

Other names Progestins; progestogens.

Most important examples
Progesterone (pregn-4-ene-3,20-dione)
17 α-hydroxyprogesterone (17 α-hydroxypregn-4-ene3,20-dione; 17 α-OHP)
20 α-hydroxyprogesterone (20 α-hydroxypregn-4-ene-3-one; 20 α-OHP; 20 α-DHP)
20 α-dihydroprogesterone; 20 α-OHP; 20 α-DHP)

Chemical characteristics Steroids with 21 carbons (C21 steroids), double bond between C4 and C5, a β-acetyl at C17 and a β-methyl at C13.

Sites of synthesis/release In women, progesterone arises from granulosa cells of ovarian follicle before ovulation; some used by theca cells for synthesis of androgens and oestrogens, though theca cells can synthesize progesterone from acetate. 17 α-OHP produced by theca interna cells of human preovulatory follicles; reaches higher plasma concentrations prior to ovulation than progesterone.

Human placenta a major source of progesterone; in other species, e.g. rabbit and goat, corpus luteum necessary as source of progesterone throughout pregnancy. Some progesterone arises from adrenal cortex.

Biosynthesis Formed by oxidation of pregnenolone which arises from acetate via cholesterol. Placenta relies on maternal blood to provide cholesterol or pregnenolone for conversion to progesterone. Progesterone a major precursor for C21 steroids, including 5 α-, 5 β-, 20 α-, and 20 β-reduced derivatives of progesterone and 17 α-OHP (an important precursor of cortisol, androgens and oestrogens).

Mechanisms of action Some actions of progestagens exerted directly on cell membranes; may form stable complexes with membrane phospholipids — perhaps basis of anaesthetic effect of progesterone, and of increase in membrane permeability to potassium which hyperpolarizes cell membranes, decreasing their excitability. Progesterone increases number and sensitivity of myometrial cell membrane β-adrenergic receptors, so making myometrium more sensitive to relaxing effects of β-adrenergic catecholamines. Inhibits development of oxytocin receptors. Stabilizes lysosomal membranes in uterine cells, so inhibiting synthesis and release of prostaglandins.

Several target tissues shown to have progesterone receptors; cytoplasmic receptor found in uterus. Activated hormone-receptor complex moves to the nucleus to affect protein synthesis etc. Progesterone decreases synthesis of oestrogen receptor protein in some uterine cells.

Physiological effects Potencies of progesterone, 17 α-OHP, and 20 α-OHP are roughly 100 per cent: 50 per cent: 5 per cent respectively. Progestagens typically hormones of pregnancy and of the luteal phase of the cycle. Progesterone most important; exerts many actions in combination with oestrogens. Regulates ovum transport through oviduct; in presence of oestrogens, depresses contractile activity of musculature of oviduct, and decreases number of cilia and secretory activity of luminal cells. Prepares uterus to receive implanting blastocyst by stimulating, with oestrogens, endometrial proliferation. Maintains pregnancy, and regulates, by disappearance from circulation at end of pregnancy, onset of parturition and lactation in some species. During pregnancy progesterone from placenta is precursor for synthesis by fetal adrenal of cortisol, corticosterone, aldosterone, and C19 androgens e.g. dehydroepiandrosterone. During menstrual cycle progesterone precipitates, by withdrawal at end of luteal phase, onset of menstruation.

Progesterone stimulates thermogenesis in women causing rise in body temperature of $0.5°C$ or less during luteal phase of cycle. Exerts mild catabolic effect, weakly mimicking corticosteroids. Binds to, but does not activate, aldosterone receptors in kidney, thus directly increases sodium excretion, but sodium retention follows because of compensatory increase in aldosterone output. Net effect, in luteal phase of cycle, is sodium and water retention.

Progesterone relaxes smooth muscle throughout body, including gall bladder and gastrointestinal tract, and especially myometrium. With oestrogens, progesterone causes growth and development of the lobular-alveolar system of mammary gland, but prevents lactogenesis because it inhibits α-lactalbumin and lactose synthesis.

Progesterone has weak anaesthetic action on brain; alters electrical activity and inhibits reflex release of oxytocin. Complex actions on secretion of anterior pituitary hormone; most important being, at high plasma concentration, to enhance *negative* feedback effect of oestradiol. High levels also block stimulatory effects of oestradiol on gonadotrophin secretion, though low levels of progesterone may *stimulate* LH release — or facilitate similar effects of oestradiol. These feedback effects exerted on anterior pituitary, on medial basal hypothalamus, and possibly on other hypothalamic areas. Progesterone also modifies behaviour: can induce sexual behaviour in ovariectomized female rat primed with oestradiol. Influences maternal behaviour: may influence nest-building in mammals, and progesterone withdrawal may contribute to onset of some behaviours of postpartum female mammal e.g. nursing, retrieving.

Progestagens cause secretion of small volumes of thick cervical mucus which can be stretched to only short distances before the thread snaps — a low 'Spinnbarkeit.' This exploited in low-dose progestagenic contraceptives which, continuously administered throughout the cycle, decrease penetrability of cervix by sperm. In certain monkeys, progesterone alters vaginal secretions so bacterial flora produce less of the aliphatic acids which enhance attractiveness of female to male.

Agonists   Several synthetic steroids have structures like natural progestagens, and are used in high- or low-dose oral contraceptives (Steele: *Gynaecology, Obstetrics and the Neonate*, Chapter 15) e.g. *norgestrel, medroxyprogesterone acetate*, and *chlormadinone acetate*. Three steroids are converted to norethisterone within body:- *lynestrenol, norethynodrel*, and *ethynodiol acetate*. Another progesterone derivative, *3α-hydroxy-5α-pregnane-11, 20-dione* ('Althesin') is a potent anaesthetic.

Antagonists   Many effects of progestagens opposed by oestrogens, but the two groups of hormones complement each other's action on many target tissues. No 'anti-progestagens' are known comparable with the anti-androgens and anti-oestrogens.

Binding   Progesterone bound to albumin (20 per cent), corticosteroid-binding globulin (CBG) (38 per cent), and to other proteins (40 per cent) leaving 2 per cent unbound. Affinity of CBG for progesterone is high, but albumin present in high concentration in plasma, so is important in progesterone binding. Bound progesterone unavailable for uptake by target cells until released in free state. CBG levels increase during pregnancy.

Disappearance rate   Progesterone distributed interchangeably in two compartments with half-lives of 2 and 15.8 minutes. Blood clearance per minute of progesterone and 17 α-OHP about 1.5 and 1.4 litres respectively.

Catabolism and excretion   Liver removes almost all progesterone it receives; uterus and mammary gland also metabolize. Metabolites include 5 α-pregnanedione, 5 β-pregnanedione, 20 α-OHP, and — the main human urinary metabolite — pregnanediol. Thirty per cent of

Prolactin

(PRL) 173

progesterone excreted as biliary conjugates of progesterone metabolites — mostly pregnanediol.

Control of release Progesterone release from granulosa cells of follicle stimulated by FSH and, when follicle well-developed, by LH. Control of progesterone release from corpus luteum varies according to species. Luteinization needs LH, but maintenance of luteal function more complex. Prolactin luteotrophic in rat, and release triggered by coitus. LH is luteotrophic in most species, including sheep, but lifespan of sheep corpus luteum determined not by luteotrophic failure, but by *luteolytic factor* (probably PGF_{2a}) from non-pregnant uterus. Placental progesterone release in human rises throughout most, or all, of gestation.

Progesterone release by sheep placenta controlled by fetal adrenal gland; rising cortisol levels at end of gestation induce activity of enzymes in placenta causing production of more oestradiol-17β and less progesterone.

Causes/effects of deficiency Short menstrual cycles may be due to lack of luteal progesterone production. Sudden withdrawal of luteal progesterone may cause premenstrual tension.

Causes/effects of excess No clinical syndrome associated with excess endogenous progesterone production. Large doses given to women in early pregnancy can be converted to androgens which masculinize genetically female fetuses.

Prolactin (PRL)

Other names Human pituitary prolactin (hPRL); lactogenic hormone.

Chemical characteristics Single chain polypeptide; 198 AAs. Mol. wt 22 554. Sequence known; similar to human growth hormone and human placental lactogen.

Site of synthesis/release From 'lactotroph' acidophilic cells in adenohypophysis. These cells rare in human pituitary except during pregnancy and lactation. Secretory granules of PRL-producing cells are irregular in size. Fetal pituitary can synthesize, store, and secrete PRL early in gestation; the process accelerates in last few weeks of gestation.

Biosynthesis By ribosomal synthesis of peptide chains.

Mechanism of action PRL-binding in cells of liver, kidney, midbrain, ovary, adrenal and seminal vesicles. Localized to the plasma membrane of mammary cells where binding of PRL induces a cAMP-dependent protein kinase; then specific proteins in plasma membranes, ribosomes and cell nuclei become phosphorylated, and specific milk proteins are induced.

Physiological effects In man, PRL has one known action — its lactogenic effect upon mammary glands. But in other species, many possible effects:

1. Nurturing of young; PRL, with other hormones, stimulates mammary growth, lactogenesis, and established milk secretion. In pigeons stimulates growth and secretion of crop 'milk'. May act on brain to stimulate maternal behaviour.

2. Gonadotrophic (and antigonadotrophic) effects: in rats PRL luteotrophic, stimulating growth and secretion of corpus luteum. At high concentrations PRL decreases ovarian steroidogenesis, and , at hypothalamo-pituitary level, diminishes oestrogen-induced LH release. Promotes vaginal mucification. On human corpus luteum, PRL may have double threshold action. Low levels needed for normal progesterone production, but high levels inhibit. PRL essential in early pregnancy and, with LH, maintains progesterone secretion.

3. Growth hormone-like effects: weak effects in males and females.

4. Osmoregulatory effects: powerful effects in teleost fish regulating water and electrolyte balance. Causes migration towards water in some fish and salamanders. In mammals, may (with aldosterone) promote renal sodium reabsorption.

5. In males may have synergistic actions with androgens on sex accessory glands.

Agonists Effects on mammary gland weakly mimicked by hPL. Pharmacological stimuli of endogenous PRL secretion by dopamine antagonists e.g. *chlorpromazine, perphenazine, reserpine, α-methyldopa, haloperidol,* and *metoclopramide*. Morphine and β-endorphin stimulate release; their effect blocked by *naloxone*. Tricyclic antidepressants e.g. *imipramine* may stimulate secretion. Oestrogen therapy promotes synthesis and release of PRL.

Antagonists   Luteotrophic effect of PRL on rat corpus luteum antagonized by PGF$_{2\alpha}$. Lactogenic effects inhibited by progesterone. Release of PRL decreased by dopamine agonists e.g. *levodopa, 2-bromo-α-ergocriptine (bromocriptine)*, and *apomorphine*. Oestrogens inhibit PRL binding to mammary tissue, and androgens inhibit PRL's action; preparations combining oestrogens and androgens used for suppression of lactation.

Binding   Some binding to plasma proteins.

Disappearance rate   Plasma half-life 20–30 minutes.

Catabolism and excretion   Liver and kidneys important in degradation.

Control of release   Maternal PRL levels rise during pregnancy; perhaps caused by rise in maternal oestrogens. Suckling stimulates release especially in early lactation. PRL released during sexual intercourse in some men and women, and by exercise or stress. PRL levels show underlying 24-hour rhythmicity, being elevated at night (i.e. during sleep).

Hypothalamus regulates PRL secretion from anterior pituitary, mainly by *prolactin release inhibiting hormone* (q.v.). PRL levels rise after pituitary stalk section. Thyrotrophin-releasing hormone (TRH) can release PRL from anterior pituitary. There may also be a distinct PRL-releasing hormone. Oestrogens increase plasma PRL levels. PRL might influence its own secretion and release through short-loop negative feedback effects on hypothalamus.

Causes/effects of deficiency   PRL deficiency rare; occurs after severe pituitary damage (e.g. in Sheehan's syndrome).

Causes/effects of excess (Steele: *Gynaecology, Obstetrics and the Neonate*, Chapters 16 and 21)   Many drugs may cause hyperprolactinaemia. Other causes include renal failure and hyperthyroidism. In about one-third of cases, hyperprolactinaemia caused by a detectable prolactin-secreting pituitary adenoma. Hyperprolactinaemia in women causes menstrual and ovulatory disorders, infertility and galactorrhoea (inappropriate lactation). Hyperprolactinaemia sometimes associated with loss of libido in men and women.

Prolactin release inhibiting hormone

Other names   Catecholamine: dopamine.

Chemical characteristics   Probably synonymous with dopamine; PRL-RIH.

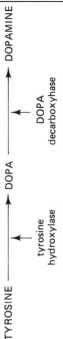

Site of synthesis/release   Dopaminergic neuron cell bodies found in medial-basal hypothalamus; axons pass to median eminence and portal vessels.

Biosynthesis   Dopamine synthesized from tyrosine:

TYROSINE $\xrightarrow{\text{tyrosine hydroxylase}}$ DOPA $\xrightarrow{\text{DOPA decarboxylase}}$ DOPAMINE

Mechanism of action   High affinity dopamine receptors in pituitary gland. Dopamine may block production, rather than release, of PRL.

Physiological effects   Dopamine reduces secretion of PRL. Dopamine important in the CNS; as a synaptic transmitter, may influence release of GnRH.

Agonists   See under PRL antagonists.

Antagonists Dopamine receptor antagonists, e.g. *metoclopramide* and *sulpiride*, induce rapid PRL release. Blockade of catecholamine synthesis by tyrosine hydroxylase inhibitor *α-methyl-p-tyrosine* increases PRL secretion. *Reserpine*, which depletes brain of dopamine, and *thyrotrophin-releasing-hormone (TRH)* stimulate PRL release.

Control of release Stimuli which stimulate (suckling, stress, oestrogens and sleep) and inhibit (PRL itself) PRL secretion probably act by exerting opposite effect on dopamine secretion into primary portal vessels.

Prostaglandins (PGs)

Chemical characteristics 20-carbon lipid-soluble unsaturated carboxylic fatty acids; two side chains joined by cyclo-pentane ring. Classified into four main groups — A, B, E, and F — according to ring substituents and number of double bonds in molecule.

Sites of synthesis/release Can be extracted from most body tissues. Low concentrations in lung, thymus, brain, kidney, umbilical cord, uterus, amniotic and menstrual fluid. Highest concentrations in seminal plasma. Seminal vesicles a major site of PG synthesis, human seminal plasma contains mainly PGE_1 and PGE_2.

Biosynthesis Synthesized in cell microsomes from essential fatty acids. Enzymes responsible found in microsomes; require molecular oxygen and a reducing agent. Bishomo-γ-linolenic acid converted to PGE_1 and/or $PGF_{1\alpha}$. Arachidonic acid, from cell membrane phospholipid, converted to PGE_2 and $PGF_{2\alpha}$ by e.g. lung, brain, endometrium, uterus, stomach. Enzyme which cleaves arachidonic acid from 2-position in phospholipid molecule — phospholipase A_2 — may control critical step in many PG-generating systems. Free arachidonic acid also present in blood plasma and may be converted through cyclo-oxygenase system to form unstable endoperoxides PGG_2 and PGH_2 (half-life in saline about 5 minutes). Endoperoxides converted by isomerase and peroxidase to PGE_2, or reduced non-enzymatically to $PGF_{2\alpha}$; also converted to unstable non-prostaglandin structures e.g. thromboxanes and prostacyclin (sometimes known as PGI_2) which have powerful effects on smooth muscle in e.g. blood vessels.

Mechanism of action/physiological effects Rapid removal of PGs from circulation, so effects normally produced in or near tissue in which they are produced i.e. they are local hormones having 'paracrine' actions. Actions of PGs of A, E, and F series often dissimilar and opposing. Profound effects on smooth muscle of e.g. intestine and uterus. PGEs depress motility of oviduct and uterus; PGFs have opposite action.

PGs are oxytocic; important in parturition. Increase free Ca^{2+} in myometrial cells, causing contraction. Can induce labour and abortion if administered intravenously in large doses or intravaginally. $PGF_{2\alpha}$ and PGE_2 present in human menstrual fluid; synthesized by endometrium and cause contractions of uterus at menstruation.

PGs (especially $PGF_{2\alpha}$) luteolytic in sheep; released from nonpregnant uterine horn, and cause regression of corpus luteum in ipsilateral ovary. May mediate induction of ovulation by LH in some species. May increase LH release acting at hypothalamic or pituitary level. Smooth muscle contractions associated with ejaculation in male not dependent on high concentrations of PGs in semen, but PGs in seminal plasma may enhance sperm transport in female tract.

PGs may be involved in implantation: *indomethacin*, the PG synthetase inhibitor, can prevent or delay implantation; $PGF_{2\alpha}$ can induce decidual response if introduced into progesterone-treated prepubertal rat.

PGs may be important in fetal haemodynamics. May regulate umbilical blood flow, especially closure of umbilical vessels after birth. Patency of ductus arteriosus attributable to PGs (probably PGEs), and postpartum closure, which has been attributed to change in oxygen tension, may be mediated by PGs or prostacyclins.

Agonists Many agents may mimic some PG actions, e.g. sympathomimetics, ergot alkaloids, and oxytocin.

Antagonists Generation of cyclic endoperoxides, the direct precursors for PG synthesis, from arachidonic acid blocked by *indomethacin* or *aspirin*, which also block prostacyclin and thromboxame production. Prostaglandin synthetase blocked by *mefenamic acid* and *ibuprofen*.

Catabolism and excretion Many PGs almost completely extracted from blood in one passage through lungs.

Control of synthesis/release In uterus synthesis of PGF_2 stimulated by oestrogens, decreased by progesterone, increased by oxytocin and by myometrial stretch. Hence sudden increase in PG production at end of pregnancy probably due mainly to increased availability of precursor, arachidonic acid; this caused by increased release of phospholipase A from ruptured lysosomes, stability of which is decreased by oestrogens and increased by progesterone. In male PG production is androgen-dependent.

Causes/effects of deficiency Concentrations of PGE in semen may be lower than normal in some cases of infertility. Women taking aspirin for rheumatoid arthritis throughout pregnancy — thereby inhibiting PG production — show prolonged gestation and increased duration of labour.

Causes/effects of excess Primary dysmenorrhoea (menstrual pains)(Steele: *Gynaecology, Obstetrics and the Neonate*, Chapter 16) may arise from excessive PG production.

Relaxin

Chemical characteristics Peptide: mol. wt about 6000. Chemical structure similar to insulin.

Site of synthesis/release Identified in human corpus luteum of pregnancy.

Physiological effects In animals (e.g. guinea pigs) relaxes ligaments of pubic symphysis. Inhibits uterine muscle contractions, so may help in maintenance of pregnancy. In human, in which the corpus luteum is not necessary for parturition, the role of relaxin is uncertain.

Further reading

Austin, C.R. and Short, R.V. (eds)(1979). *Mechanisms of Hormone Action.* Book 7 of *Reproduction in Mammals.* Cambridge University Press, Cambridge.

Bentley, P.J. (1980). *Endocrine Pharmacology.* Cambridge University Press, Cambridge.

Beyer, C. (ed.)(1979). *Comprehensive Endocrinology: Endocrine Control of Sexual Behavior.* Raven Press, New York.

Franchimont, P. and Channing, C. (eds)(1981). *Intragonadal Regulation of Reproduction.* Academic Press, London.

Greep, R.O. (ed.)(1973). *Female Reproductive System.* Parts 1 and 2 of Volume II of Section 7 (Endocrinology) of the American Handbook of Physiology. American Physiological Society, Washington, D.C.

Ismail, A.A.A. (1981). *Biochemical Investigations in Endocrinology.* Academic Press, London.

Schulster, D.S., Burstein, S. and Cooke, B.A. (1976). *Molecular Endocrinology of the Steroid Hormones.* John Wiley, London.

Index

Abortion 72
ABP *see* Androgens, binding protein
Acrosin 66
Acrosome 56, 59, 65-6
ACTH *see* Adrenocorticotrophic hormone
Activation of spermatozoa 65-6
Adenohypophysis *see* Pituitary
Adipose tissue 14, 125
Adolescent growth spurt 13-14
Adrenal cortex
  androgens 17-18, 47, 62, 119-21, 136, 160
  fetal 118-22, 136
  hypoplasia 122, 136, 170
  lactogenesis 142, 143
  maturation at puberty 17-18
  parturition 136
  pregnant mother 85
  stress 22
Adrenaline 75, 122-3
Adrenal medulla 122, 123
Adrenarche 17-18, 161
Adrenocorticotrophic hormone (ACTH) 118-19, 136, 143
Adrenogenital syndrome 3, 10, 12
Albumin 81, 92
Alcohol 82, 101
Aldosterone 46, 86, 112, 119, 121, 157
Aliphatic acids and sexual behaviour 20, 46
Allantoic cavity 113
Allantois 4
Allergies 92
Allometric growth 140
Alpha-fetoprotein 114
Amenorrhoea 83, 152, 163, 167
Amino acids 80, 81, 87, 110
Amniocentesis 114
Amniochorion 112, 114
Amniotic cavity 69, 113
Amniotic fluid 112-16
  collection 114
  composition 114-16
  cortisol levels 122
  discharge during labour 131
  excess (polyhydramnios) 114
  fetal kidney 111, 112
  fetal skin 112, 113
  formation 112, 113-14
  hPL 114, 165
  insufficient (oligohydramnios) 114
  osmotic pressure 114, 115

prolactin 116
pulmonary surfactant 114
volume change 97-8, 113
water 86, 88
Ampulla *see* Oviducts ampulla
Amygdala 17, 20, 24, 27
Anabolic steroids 161
Androgens 160-62
adrenal
  female libido 47, 62
  fetal 119-21, 136
  parturition 136
  puberty 17-18
agonists 161
antagonists 10-11, 47, 61, 161
aromatization 11, 35-6, 119-20, 157, 160, 168, 169
binding in blood 161
binding in brain 27
binding protein (ABP) 52-3, 58, 160
biosynthesis 52, 120, 157, 160
catabolism and excretion 161
control of release 161
  adrenal cortex at puberty 17-18
  fetus 7, 117
  ovary 36
  testis 53
  theca interna of follicle 36
deficiency 3, 8-9, 161-2
effects 160-61
  activational 11
  behaviour 61
  organizational 10-11
  prostaglandin production 176
  sperm maturation 58-9
  spermatogenesis 57, 58
excess 3, 10, 11, 12, 162
fetal 3, 10, 119-20, 136
follicular synthesis 35-6
levels 41, 158
mechanism of action 160
menopause 47
ovarian 36, 47
receptors 9, 52, 58
synthesis in
  fetal adrenal cortex 119-20, 136, 160
  ovarian follicle 35-6, 160
  target tissues 7-9, 58-9, 160
  testis 52-3, 159, 160

testicular 52-3, 57, 58-9
  see also Testosterone
Androstenedione 160-62
  biosynthesis 157
  chemical formula 120, 157
  feto-placental unit 120
  levels 41, 158
  secretion in puberty 17
  synthesis by follicle 35-6
Anencephaly 114, 116; 118, 136
Aneupolidy 1-4
Angiotensin II 46, 75
Anorexia nervosa 21, 163, 164, 167
Anti-androgens, *see* Androgens, Cyproterone acetate
Antibodies 90-94
  maternal 92
Antigen
  fetal 89, 92
  H-Y 4
  HLA 92
  inoculation with 94
  paternal 89-90
  rhesus 92
Arachidonic acid 135, 175, 176
Areola 140, 141
Aspirin 176
Atresia, oesophageal 114
Auditory stimuli 21
Auto-immune reactions 94
Autosomes 1

Barr body 1, 2
Basal lamina 33, 34
Behaviour
  aggressive 160
  ante-natal 153-4
  maternal 153-5
  menopausal changes 48
  menstrual cycle 46-7
  nest building 153-4
  parturition, during 154
  post partum 154-5
  pregnancy 89
  sexual 10-11, 20, 43, 46-7, 61-4, 160, 161, 169
Beta-lipotrophin 119
Beta-melanocyte-stimulating hormone (β-MSH) 119
Bifidus factor 151
Bilirubin 109-10
  amniotic fluid 116
  encephalopathy 109
Biliverdin 109
Birds, control of egg-laying 17, 20-21

Birth canal 131
Bladder 7–8, 50, 87
Blastocyst 67–72, 83
Blindness, and onset of puberty 12, 20
Block to polyspermy 37, 66–7
Blood pressure in pregnancy 86–7
Blood-testis barrier 52
Blood volume
  fetal 104–5
  maternal 86
  neonatal, and jaundice 110
B lymphocytes 90
Bohr *see* Double Bohr effect
Bonding 154–5
Bone
  androgens and 14, 160–61
  menopause 47, 170
  oestrogens and 14, 47, 169, 170
  puberty 14
Bottle feeding 94, 145
Breast
  blood supply 140, 141
  cancer 139, 140
  development
    postnatal 139–40
    pregnancy 141–2
    puberty 13–14, 140
  feeding 89, 94, 110, 139, 145, 149–52, 155
  involution after menopause 47, 153
  lymphatic drainage 140
  menstrual cycle, changes during 140, 141
  Montgomery's glands 140
  myoepithelial cells 140, 141, 144–5, 146
  nerve supply 140–41
  nipple 62, 63, 140, 141, 142, 146
  sexual response 62, 63, 139
  structure in adult 140–41
  tactile sensitivity 141
  see also Lactation, Mammary glands, Milk
Bromocriptine 144, 174
Brown adipose tissue (BAT) 125–6
Bruce effect 20
Bulbourethral (Cowper's) glands 7–8, 50, 60

Calcium 65, 80, 81, 132, 149, 150
Cancer
  breast 12, 139, 140
  choriocarcinoma 75, 164
  prostate 60
Capacitation of spermatozoa 64–5
Carbon dioxide 70, 76–9
Carbonic anhydrase 79
Carboxyhaemoglobin 100
Cardiac output
  pregnant mother 86
Cardiovascular system
  pregnant mother 86–7
Carotid body chemoreceptors 106–8
Casein 149, 150
Catecholamines 24–7
Catecholoestrogens 26–7

CBG *see* Cortisol-binding globulin
Central nervous system
  fetal 127–8
  menstrual cycle 35, 39, 42–3, 46–7
  pregnancy 89
  puberty 14–17
Cerebral palsy 126
Cerebrospinal fluid (CSF) 24–5, 127, 163
Cervix, uterine
  compliance 133
  connective tissue 133
  effacement 130, 133
  menopause 47
  menstrual cycle 45–6
  mucus 45–6, 64
  mucus plug 130
  oestrogens and 45–6, 64, 133, 168
  parturition 130–31, 133, 135
  pregnancy, changes during 130, 133
  progestagens and 64, 172
  prostaglandins and 133, 135
  structure 30
Chemoreceptors 106, 107–8
Chimpanzee 18, 118
Chlormadinone acetate 172
Christiansen-Douglas-Haldane effect 79
Chromosomes
  abnormalities 1–5
  fertilization 67
  sex 1–5, 7
  sperm formation 53
  X and Y 1–5, 7, 50
Cholesterol 81, 119–20, 157, 160, 168, 171
Choriocarcinoma 75, 164
Chorion 136
Circadian rhythms 19
Circumventricular organs 24–5
Cleavage 67, 68
Climacteric 47–8, 163
CLIP *see* Corticotrophin-like intermediate lobe peptide
Clitoris 7, 9, 62, 63
Clomiphene 166, 169
Coitus
  description 62, 63, 64
  interruptus 63
  ovulation 21, 43, 62, 164
  prolactin release 21
Colostrum 91, 93, 94, 140, 142, 149, 150
Conjugation, steroids 81–2
Contraception
  breast-feeding, effect of 139, 152
  coitus interruptus 63
  intrauterine device (IUD) 72
  'mini-pills' 64, 172
  'morning after pills' 170
  oestrogens 169
  oral contraceptives 169, 172
  post-coital 170
  progestagens 64, 172
  steroid 163, 166, 169, 170, 172
Contractions, uterine
  labour 130–33, 152
  menstrual cycle 45
  sexual response 63

Copulation *see* Coitus
Corona radiata 34
Coronary thrombosis 12, 47, 169
Corpus albicans 31
Corpus cavernosum of the penis 7, 50, 63
Corpus luteum
  formation 31, 38
  human chorionic gonadotrophin 39, 40, 43, 71, 83
  luteinizing hormone 38
  luteolysis 38–40, 71, 83, 173, 175
  maintenance 38–40, 71–2; 83, 164, 173
  oestrogen secretion 38
  pregnancy 38–40, 71–2, 83, 133–4
  progestagen secretion 38
Cortex, of gonad 4
Corticosteroids 22, 106, 110, 119–23, 141, 143
Corticosterone 119, 121, 157
Corticotrophin-like intermediate lobe peptide (CLIP) 119
Cortical cords 5
Cortical vesicles 37, 66–7
Cortisol
  biosynthesis 121, 157
  effects
    fetal lung 106
    lactogenesis 142, 144
    mammary gland growth 140
    neonatal carbohydrate metabolism 127
    onset of parturition in sheep 122, 136
  fetal adrenal 119, 121
Cortisol-binding-globulin (CBG) 85, 86, 143, 144
Cortisone 122, 157
Cowper's (bulbourethral) gland 7–8, 50, 60
Creatinine 81, 111, 114, 115
Cretinism 118
Crista dividens 101
Cryptorchidism 51
CSF *see* Cerebrospinal fluid
Cumulus oophorus 34, 36, 65
Curd 149
Cyproterone 161
Cyproterone acetate 11, 47, 61, 161
Cysteine 111
Cystine 80, 111
Cytotrophoblast 69, 70, 74, 164

Decidua (-lization) 70, 74, 122, 135
Defeminization 10-12
  see also Pseudohermaphroditism
Dehydroepiandrosterone (DHEA) 47, 119–20, 157, 160–61
  sulphate 119–20, 136, 161
Deoxyribonucleic acid (DNA) 33, 53, 67, 141, 142
DHA *see* Dehydroepiandrosterone
DHEA *see* Dehydroepiandrosterone

DHT *see* 5α-Dihydro-
    testosterone
Diabetes 85, 99, 124, 125, 127
Diethylstilboestrol 169
Differentiation, sexual *see*
    Sexual differentiation
20α-Dihydroprogesterone
    see 20α-Hydroxyprogesterone
5α-Dihydrotestosterone (DHT)
    157-62
    biosynthesis 157
    chemical formula 157
    effects 160
    epididymis 58-9
    sexual differentiation 7-9
Dimethylstilboestrol 169
Dipalmitoyl-lecithin (DPL) 106,
    114, 123
2,3 Diphosphoglycerate (DPG)
    77
DNA *see* Deoxyribonucleic acid
Donne bodies 142
Dopamine
    appearance in hypothalamus
        116
    GnRH 164
    nerve cells and fibres 24
    synthesis, inhibition by cate-
        choloestrogens 27
    see also Prolactin release
        inhibiting hormone
Double Bohr effect 77
Down's syndrome 116, 170
DPG *see* 2,3 Diposphoglycerate
DPL *see* Dipalmitoyl-lecithin
Drugs
    fetal growth 101
    in milk 151
    placental transfer 82
Ducts
    Müllerian (paramesonephric)
        6-9
    Wolffian (mesonephric) 7-8
Ductus arteriosus 101, 102,
    103, 104, 105, 176
Ductus venosus 101, 102
Dysmenorrhoea 176
Dyspareunia 47

E₁ *see* Oestrone
E₂ *see* Oestradiol
E₃ *see* Oestriol
Ectopic pregnancy 67
Effacement of cervix 130, 133
Ejaculation 50, 61, 63, 64
Embryo
    early development 67-70
    implantation 69-72
    transport 67
Endometrium *see* Uterus
    endometrium
β-Endorphin 173
Environment, external 19-22,
    57, 61-2, 137
Ependymal tanycytes *see*
    Tanycytes
Epididymis 7-8, 50-51, 57-9,
    160
Epithelium, germinal 4-5
Ergometrine 170
Ergonovine 170
Erogenous zones 62
Erythrocytes 75
Erythrocyte sedimentation rate
    86

Erythropoiesis, fetal 79
Escherichia coli 94, 150, 151
Eupolidy 2
Exaltolide 20

Facilitated diffusion 76, 80, 81
Fallopian tube, *see* Oviduct
Fat
    fetal accumulation 97, 125
    maternal deposition in
        pregnancy 88-9
    maternal metabolism 87
    milk 147-8, 150
Free fatty acids, placental
    transport 81-2
Feedback
    negative
        male 53, 57-8
        puberty 14-17
        menstrual cycle 35, 39,
            41-3
    milk secretion, control of
        144
    oestradiol 168
    positive 36, 42, 137, 168-9
Fertility 21
Fertilization 33, 45, 64-8
Feto-placental unit 6, 119-22,
    136, 170
Fetus, fetal 96-128
    abnormalities of head 136
    acid-base balance 132
    adrenal cortex 118-23, 136,
        170
    adrenal medulla 122, 123
    adrenalectomy 136
    adrenocorticotrophic
        hormone (ACTH)
        118-19, 136
    alcohol syndrome 101
    aldosterone 119, 121
    amniotic fluid 113-116
    anencephaly 114, 116, 118,
        136
    bilirubin 109-10
    blood-brain barrier 127
    blood pressure 111
    brain
        blood supply 106
        damage 109, 126, 132
        drugs 128
        ketone body utilization
            127
        masculinization 10-12,
            169
        metabolism 127
        reflexes 128
        'breathing' 106
    calcium levels 124
    central nervous system
        127-8
    cerebrospinal fluid 127
    chemoreceptors 106, 107-8
    circulation 73, 101-5
    corticosteroids 106, 119-23,
        126, 136
    cortisol 106, 119, 121-22,
        126, 136
    death in utero 136
    dipalmitoyl lecithin 106, 114,
        123
    endocrinology 116-24
    erythropoiesis 79
    fat deposition 125
    fatty acid levels 125

feto-placental unit 119-22,
    136
follicle stimulating hormone
    6, 117, 118
fluids *see* Amniotic fluid
gastrointestinal tract 112,
    114
glucagon 124, 126
glucose levels 124
glycogen, liver 123, 126
gonadotrophins 6, 117
gonads 4-9, 117-18
growth 96-101
    anencephaly 116
    cigarette smoking 100
    drugs 101
    fetal damage 98
    fetal hormones 99
    fetal kidney 111
    human growth hormone
        116
    hypophysectomy 116
    maternal age 100
    maternal alcohol
        consumption 101
    maternal diabetes 99,
        124
    maternal heart disease
        100
    maternal hypertension
        100
    maternal nutrition 100
    maternal size 99
    multiple pregnancy 99
    placenta 99, 100
    racial differences 98
    sex of fetus 99
    socio-economic factors
        100
    heart 101-3
    heart rate during labour
        131-2
    hormones 6, 116-24
    human chorionic
        gonadotrophin 6, 117
    human chorionic thyro-
        trophin 118
    human growth hormone 116
    hyperglycaemia 124, 132
    hypoglycaemia 106
    hypophysectomy 116, 136
    hypothalamic-pituitary axis
        116, 118
    hypoxia 106, 132
    immunoglobulins 90-94
        synthesis 91-2
    infection 91-2, 94
    insulin 124
    kidney 111
        amniotic fluid 111,
            112, 113
    lactate accumulation 132
    lipid metabolism 125
    lipogenesis 124
    liver 109-10, 122, 123,
        126-7
    lungs 103, 106, 112, 114,
        122, 125
    lung surfactant 106
    luteinizing hormone 6, 117,
        118
    membranes 74, 112, 122,
        130, 131, 134, 135
    myocardium 122
    oestradiol 6, 11, 117-18

origin from blastocyst 67
ovary 117–18
pancreas 123–4
parathormone 124
phospholipids 125
physiology during labour
131–2
pituitary gland 116–17,
118–19, 126, 136
prolactin 116–17, 118
pulmonary circulation 101,
103, 105
reflexes 128
respiratory movements 106
respiratory tract 106, 112
reverse tri-iodothyronine 118
sexing in utero 1
skin 112, 113
spelling vi
spleen 92
stomach 113
sympathetic activation 107
testes 4–9, 117
testosterone 6–8, 117
thyroid gland 99, 118
thyroxine 81, 118
triglyceride levels 125
tri-iodothyronine 118
urinary tract 112
urine 111, 113
vascular channels 101
vasopressin 123
vitamin D and derivatives
124
zone, of adrenal cortex 118,
122, 136
Fibrinogen 86
Fick's Law 76–7
Fimbria *see* Oviduct fimbria
Fœtus *see* Fetus
Follicles *see* Ovarian follicles
Follicle stimulating hormone
(FSH) 162–3
catabolism and excretion 162
chemical characteristics 162
control of release 162–3
external environment
19–22
female cycle 39–43
GnRH 162
inhibin 39, 42, 163,
165–6
male 57, 58
neural 22–7
post-menopausal 47, 48
puberty 14–17
effects 162
follicular development
and steroidogenesis
35–6, 162, 170
mechanism of 162
spermatogenesis 57, 162
levels 158
fetus 6, 117
menopause 47–8
menstrual cycle 39–42,
48
puberty 14–17, 48, 158
receptors 35–6, 57, 58
synthesis 39, 162
Follicular phase *see* Ovary cycle
Foramen ovale 101, 102, 104,
105
FSH *see* Follicle stimulating
hormone

Galactopoiesis 144, 145
Galactorrhoea 173
Galactosyl transferase 142, 147,
148
Gametes 1, 67
see also Oocyte, Spermatozoa
Gastroenteritis 150
Gender identity 12
Genetics of sex 1–5
Genital primordia 4–9
Genitalia
differentiation 6–10, 160
female, structure 29
male, structure 50–51
sexual response 63
Germ cells
female, life cycle 33
male 53
see also Primordial germ cells
Germinal epithelium 4–5
Germinal vesicle 32, 37
Glans penis 7, 9, 50
Glucagon 110, 124, 127
Glucose
hPL effects on metabolism of
85
levels 124, 126–7, 132
milk synthesis 147, 148
placental transport 80, 81
pregnant mother 85, 87
testis tubule fluid 52
Glucuronyl transferase 109, 110
Glycerol, milk synthesis 148
Glycogen 122, 126
Glycogen synthetase 126
Glycosaminogylcans 133
GnRH *see* Gonadotrophin
releasing hormone
Gonads 4–7
see also Ovary, Testis
Gonadotrophins
control 39–43, 139
levels 158
menopause 47–8
menstrual cycle 39–43
puberty 14–17
role in follicular development
35–7
suppression by suckling 139
Gonadotrophin releasing
hormone (GnRH) 163–4
appearance in hypothalamus
116, 162
catabolism and excretion 163
chemical characteristics 163
control of release 163–4
effects 163
LH surge 21, 39, 42–3
menstrual cycle, role in
39, 42–3
half-life 163
nerve cells and fibres 24–5
secretion during puberty
14–17
Graafian follicle 34, 163
Granulosa cells 32, 34–8, 167, 173
Growth hormone *see* Human
growth hormone
'Guevedoces' 3–9
Gynaecomastia 140
Gynandromorphs 4

Haematocrit 86
Haemoglobin
adult 77–8

catabolism 109
concentration
adult/fetal difference
77–8
male/female difference 12
fetal 77–8
Haemolytic disease of the
newborn 75, 116
Haemorrhoids 88
hCG *see* Human chorionic
gonadotrophin
hCS *see* Human placental
lactogen
hCT *see* Human chorionic
thyrotrophin
Head's paradoxical inflation
reflex 108
Hering-Breuer inflation reflex
108
Hermaphrodites 4, 12
Heroin 128
Hippocampus 20, 24
Histamine 70, 75
Histidine 87
hMG *see* Human menopausal
gonadotrophin
Homosexuality 12, 62–4
Hormones (*see under* individual
hormones)
binding in brain 27
definition 20
levels 158–9
fetus 6
menopause 48
menstrual cycle 41
pregnancy 84
placental transport 81
hPL *see* Human placental
lactogen
Human chorionic
gonadotrophin (hCG)
164–5
amniotic fluid 114
effects 164
fetal testis 6–7, 14–16,
52, 117, 161, 164
immunological 90, 164
luteotrophic 39, 40, 43,
71, 83, 164
levels
fetus 6, 117
pregnant mother 84
placental transfer 81
Human chorionic somatomammotrophin (hCS) *see*
Human placental lactogen
Human chorionic thyrotrophin
85
Human growth hormone
(hGH) 116, 140, 143
Human menopausal gonado-
trophin (hMG) 166
Human placental lactogen
(hPL) 165
amniotic fluid 114
effects 165
breast development 141,
143, 165
immunological 85, 90,
165
lactogenesis 142, 143
metabolic 85, 87, 165
levels 84
placental transfer, lack of 81,
165

source 83, 85
Hyaline membrane disease
    (HMD) 106
H-Y antigen 4
Hyaluronidase 65
Hydramnios 114
16α-Hydroxydehydroepi-
    androsterone sulphate
    119–20, 157
17α-Hydroxyprogesterone 121,
    157, 171–3
    biosynthesis 120–21, 157
    by feto-placental unit
        120–21
    luteal 38
    menopause 47
    stimulation of LH release 42
20α-Hydroxyprogesterone
    171–3
Hyperbilirubinaemia 110
Hyperglycaemia 124, 132
Hyperkalaemia 112
Hyperprolactinaemia 174
Hypernatraemia 151
Hypertension, maternal 100
Hypertyrosinaemia 111
Hyperventilation 131
Hypoglycaemia 106, 110, 123,
    124, 126–7
Hyponatraemia 112
Hypophysectomy 116
Hypothalamus 22–7
    anatomical features 22–3
    connexions 20, 22, 24
    development 116
    ependymal tanycytes 24
    hypophysiotrophic area 22
    lactogenesis, role in 143
    magnocellular neurosecretory
        system 24
    masculinization 10-11
    menstrual cycle 35, 39–43
    parvicellular neurosecretory
        system 24
    pituitary 14–18, 19, 22–4,
        27, 43, 116
    puberty 14–18, 43
    sexual behaviour 10-11, 46
    site of hormone feedback
        14–16, 42–3
    suprachiasmatic nucleus 19,
        164
    temperature set-point 46
    see also Feedback
Hypoxia 103, 104, 106, 132

ICSH *see* Luteinizing hormone
Idiopathic respiratory distress
    syndrome (IRDS) 106,
    122
Immunological paralysis 94
Immunological tolerance 94
Immunology of pregnancy 73,
    75, 89–94
Immunoglobulins (Ig)
    fetal 90–93
    IgA 91–4
        secretory 91, 94, 141,
            147, 149–50
    IgD 91, 92
    IgE 92
    IgG 91–4, 149
    IgM 91–2, 93, 94
    levels after birth 93–4

placental transport 81, 91,
    92
Implantation 39, 40, 69–72, 73,
    83, 168, 176
Impotence 22, 61, 161, 163,
    167
Infundibulum *see* Oviduct
    infundibulum
Inhibin 165–166
    follicular 39, 42
    testicular 57, 58
Inner cell mass 67
Insulin 85, 87, 124, 127, 140,
    141, 142
Interstitial cell stimulating
    hormone (ICSH) *see*
    Luteinizing hormone
Involution, mammary 152–3
Iodide 80
IRDS *see* Idiopathic respiratory
    distress syndrome
Iron 80, 81
IUD *see* Contraception,
    intrauterine device

Jaundice, neonatal 110

Kallman's syndrome 163, 164,
    167
Kernicterus 109
Ketone bodies 125, 127
Klinefelter's syndrome 2–3

Labia, majora and minora 7, 9,
    14, 63
Labour, *see* Parturition
α-Lactalbumin 142, 147, 148
Lactation 139-155
    cessation 152–3
    during pregnancy 153
    effects on mother 151–2
    effect on mother–infant
        relationship 152
    energy provision 89, 151–2
    failure 128, 144
    fertility during 21, 139, 152,
        153
    importance of 139, 149–52
    inappropriate (galactorrhoea)
        174
    lactogenesis 142 .
    weaning 127, 153
    see also Breast, Mammary
        gland, Milk
Lactobacillus 150–51
Lactoferrin 149–50, 151
Lactogenesis 142–4, 172
β-Lactoglobulin 148, 149
Lactose synthetase 142, 147,
    148
Lactotroph 85
Laryngeal changes at puberty
    14
Lee-Boot effect 20
Leydig cells *see* Testis interstitial
    cells
LH *see* Luteinizing hormone
Libido
    control
        men 61–2
        women 47, 61–2
    hyperprolactinaemia 174
    menopause 48
Life expectancy, male/female 12
Ligandin 109–10

Light 12, 19–20, 24–5, 164
Lipids
    fetal metabolism 125
    placental transfer 81–2
Liquor
    amnii *see* Amniotic fluid
    folliculi 34
Lordosis 10–11
Low birth weight 96, 100, 127
Lungs
    fetal/neonatal 101, 103, 104,
        106–7
    pregnant mother 87
Luteal phase *see* Ovary cycle
Luteinizing hormone (LH)
    166–7 ·
    chemical characteristics 166
    control of release 166–7
    coitus-induced 43
    external environment
        19–21
    GnRH 42–3, 163, 166
    hypothalamus 11, 17,
        39–43, 166–7
    male 53
    menstrual cycle 39–43
    oestrogens 11, 166
    progesterone 165
    puberty 14–17
    corpus luteum 38, 40
    effects 166
    ovarian 35–8, 166, 170
    spermatogenesis 57, 58,
        166
    stimulation of androgen
        production 57, 58,
            161, 166
    follicular development 35–8
    half-life 166
    levels 157
        fetus 6, 117
        menopause 47–8
        menstrual cycle 41
    menstrual cycle 35–43
    puberty 14–17, 20
    receptors 35–7, 57–8, 166
    surge 10–11, 19, 37, 39–43
    synthesis 39
Luteinizing hormone releasing
    hormone (LHRH, LRF),
    see Gonadotrophin-
    releasing hormone
    (GnRH)
Luteolysis 38–40, 71, 83, 173
Lymph nodes 90, 91
Lysosomes 135
Lysozyme (muramidase) 150

Magnocellular neurosecretory
    system 24
Mammary gland
    development 14, 139–40
    immunoglobulin synthesis 94
    involution 152–3
    lactogenesis 142–4
    oestrogens, effect of 140,
        141, 169
    secretory mechanisms 145–9
    ultrastructure of secretory
        cell 147
    see also Breast, Lactation,
        Milk
Masculinization 7–12
    see also Pseudoherma-
        phroditism

Masturbation 61
Maternal behaviour 128, 139, 153–5
Maternal physiology
  labour 131
  pregnancy 83–9
Medulla, of gonad 4
Meiosis 1
  oocyte 32–3, 37, 67
  spermatocyte 53–4
Melatonin 25
Membrana propria 33
Menarche 12, 16
  see also Puberty
Menopause 47–8, 153, 158–9, 163, 166, 170
Menstrual cycle
  changes in
    brain and behaviour 46–7
    breasts 46, 140, 141
    cervix 45–6
    ovary 29–39
    endometrium 44–5
    hormone levels 41, 158–9
    myometrium 45
    oviduct 45
    vagina 46
  control 39–43
  definition 29
  duration 31–2, 39
  synchronization 20
Menstruation 29, 32, 41, 44–5
Mesonephric ducts, see Wolffian ducts
Mesonephros 8, 111
Metabolic changes in pregnancy 87
Metanephros 111
Methadone 128
Methionine 111
Micturition 87
Milk
  accumulation in breast 144
  bifidus factor 151
  composition 111, 149–51
  effect of 125, 149–51
  electrolytes 148–9
  fat 147–8, 149
  immunoglobulins 91, 93, 94, 141, 146, 149, 150
  lactoferrin 49–50, 151
  lactose 126, 142, 147, 148, 150
  lysozyme 150
  output volume 149
  phosphate 150, 151
  potassium 148, 150
  protein 145, 147, 149–50
  secretion
    cellular mechanisms 145–9
    cessation 152–3
    energy needs 151–2
    initiation see Lactogenesis
    regulation by demand 144–5
    maintenance see Galacto-poiesis
  sodium 148, 150
  toxic substances 151
  vitamins 149, 150, 151
  water 148, 149
  witches' 140

Milk ejection reflex 144–6
  fat composition of milk, and 149
  inhibition of 144, 145–6
  neuroendocrine mechanisms 21
  stimulation of reproductive tract 146
  stress 21, 144
  suckling 144, 146
Mitosis 32–3, 52–4, 89
Monkey
  control of gonadotrophins 42, 167
  fetal adrenal cortex 118
  pregnancy termination 85
  sexual interaction 20, 22, 62
Montgomery's glands 140
'Morning after pills' 170
Morning sickness 89
Morphine 128, 173
Morula 67, 68
Mosaics 4
Mounting behaviour 10–11
Mucus, cervical 45–6, 64
Müllerian inhibiting hormone 6–7, 10, 167
Myoepithelial cells 140, 141, 144–5, 146
Myometrium See Uterus myometrium

Naloxone 173
Natural childbirth 137
Neonate, neonatal
  ACTH 119
  adrenal cortex 122
  adrenaline 122, 123
  aldosterone 112, 122
  anoxia 77
  auto-immune reactions 94
  brain damage 111, 126
  brain metabolism 127
  breathing 105–8
    acidosis 107
    apnoea 108
    asphyxia 107, 127
    auditory stimuli
    chemoreceptors 107–8
    cooling 108
    Head's paradoxical inflation reflex 108
    Hering-Breuer inflation reflex 108
    immersion 108
    lung stretch receptors 108
    opiates 108
    painful stimuli 108
    release from obtunded state 108
    sympathetic activation 107, 108
    tactile stimulation 108
  brown adipose tissue 125–6
  calcium levels 124
  carbohydrate metabolism 126–7
  circulation 103–5
    control mechanisms 105
    ductus arteriosus 104
    foramen ovale 105
    placental transfusion 104–5

pulmonary vascular resistance 103, 104, 105, 107
  ventricles, size of 105
  corticosterone 122
  cortisol 122, 127
  endocrinology 116–24
  fatty acid levels 125
  follicle stimulating hormone 48, 117
  glucagon 126, 127
  glucose levels 126–7
  glycogen stores, liver 127
  gut acidity 150–51
  heat production 126
  hyperinsulinaemia 124
  hypernatraemia 151
  hypocalcaemia 151
  hypoglycaemia 110, 123, 124, 126–7
  hypothyroid 99
  hypoxia 108
  immunoglobulins 92–4
  inoculation 94
  insulin 126, 127
  iron 151
  ketone bodies 125, 127
  kidney 111–12
  liver 109–10, 125, 126
  lung 105–8
  luteinizing hormone 48, 117
  mammary glands 140
  non-shivering thermogenesis 126
  nutrition 152
    see also Milk
  oxytocin 123
  pancreas 126
  parathormone 124
  prolactin 117
  respiratory distress syndrome 106, 122
  sex-hormone binding globulin 117
  sleep 127–8
  sodium, excretion and retention 112, 151
  suckling, depression of 145
  swallowing 108
  testosterone 117
  thermoregulation 125–6
  thyrocalcitonin 124
  thyroid deficiency 118
  thyroid stimulating hormone 118
  thyroxine 127
  triglyceride levels 125
  uraemia 151
  urea excretion 112
  urine flow 111, 112
  vitamin D 151
  vitamin K 82
  water retention 151
Nest building 89, 153–4
Neuroendocrinology 22–7
  menstrual cycle 39–43, 46–7
  puberty 14–18
Neurohypophysis, see Pituitary, posterior
Neurophysin 170
Newborn babies see Neonate
Non-disjunction, maternal and paternal 2
Noradrenaline 25–6, 75, 116, 122–3, 125, 164

Nucleus
 sexually dimorphic 11
 suprachiasmatic 19, 22–4, 43
Nutrition 12, 21, 89, 94, 163
Nycthemeral rhythms 19

Oedema 86, 87
Oesophageal atresia 114
Oestradiol 167–70
 biosynthesis 35–7, 119–20,
  157
 chemical formula 120, 157
 implantation 70
 levels 159
  fetal 6, 82, 117–18
  menstrual cycle 41
  pregnant mother 82, 84
 menstrual cycle 35–43
 neonatal injections, effects
  11
 receptors 36, 44
 stimulation of LH release
  42, 168–9
 uterus 44–5
 see also Oestrogens
Oestriol 167–70
 biosynthesis 119–20, 157
 chemical formula 120, 157
 levels 82, 84, 119
Oestrogens 167–70
 antagonists 169
 binding in brain 27
 binding protein 27
 catabolism and excretion 169
 catecholoestrogens 26–7
 chemical characteristics 157,
  167
 control of release 36, 170
 effects 168–9
  behaviour 20, 43, 46–7,
   62
  bone 47
  breast development 140
  cervix 45–6, 168
  endometrium 44–5, 168,
   170
  gonadotrophin release
   42, 168–9
  implantation 70–72
  lactogenesis 142, 143
  lysosomal instability 135
  mammary gland 140,
   142–4, 168
  masculinization 11
  metabolic 87
  myometrium 132–3,
   135, 168
  oviduct 45
  prolactin release 142–3,
   169, 174
  prostaglandin synthesis
   122, 135, 176
  'protective' in fetus 117
  side effects 170
  uterus 44–5, 71–2, 75,
   132–3, 168
  vagina 20, 46–7, 168
 impeded oestrogens 169
 levels 159
  fetal 6, 82
  menstrual cycle 41
  pregnant mother 82, 84
 menopause 47
 menstrual cycle 35–43

placental transport 81–2
 synthesis 157, 167–8
 feto-placental unit
  119–20, 136
 follicle 35–7
Oestrone 167–70
 biosynthesis 120, 157
 chemical formula 120, 157
 levels 41, 82, 84, 159
Oestrous cycle 10–11
 control 43
 definition 29
Oestrous behaviour 29, 43, 46
Olfactogenital syndrome see
  Kallman's syndrome
Olfactory stimuli 20, 43, 47,
  144, 164, 168
Oligohydramnios 114
Oocyte
 chromosomes 1
 fertilization 65–7
 formation 4–5
 follicular development 31
 lifespan 65
 meiosis 32–3, 37
 numbers 32
 primary 32–3
 secondary 33, 37
 sperm penetration 33
 transport 65
Oogonia 4, 32
Organum vasculosum of the
  lamina terminalis
  (OVLT) 24–5, 163
Orgasm 61, 63
Osteoporosis after menopause
  47, 170
Ovary (ovarian)
 control
  environment 19–22
  neural 22–7
  pituitary hormones
   33–43, 162, 166
  puberty 14–17
  uterus 38–40, 43
 cycle
  duration 31–2, 39
  hormone levels 41, 158–9
  follicular phase 39, 41,
   71
  luteal phase 31, 38–39,
   41, 71
 development 4–5, 7, 32–3
 failure in menopause 47
 follicles 29, 31–8
  androgen synthesis 35–6
  antral 34
  atresia 31–2, 36
  development 32–8
  dominance 36
  fetal 118
  fluid 34, 36
  inhibin 39, 42
  oestrogen synthesis
   35–6, 167
  ovulation 31, 37–8
  preantral 32–6
  preovulatory 37
  primary, secondary and
   tertiary 33–4, 36
  primordial 32, 34
  progesterone synthesis
   35, 173
  stigma 37
 germ cells, numbers 32, 47

lactogenesis, role in 143
 oestrogens, effect of 169
 stromal tisue 32, 34
 structure 29–31
Oviducts (Fallopian tubes)
  29–30
 ampulla 30, 64, 65
 cilia 67
 development 7–9
 embryo transport 67, 68, 72
 fimbria 30, 38, 64
 infundibulum 30
 isthmus 65, 67
 menopause 47
 menstrual cycle 45
 musculature 67
 oestrogens 45
 oocyte transport 65, 72
 ostium 38
 progestagens 45, 67, 172
 sperm transport 64–5
 tubal pregnancy 67
OVLT see Organum
  vasculosum of the lamina
  terminalis
Ovotestis 4
Ovulation
 definition 29
 mechanism 37–8
 oocyte 33
 reflex 21, 29, 43, 62
 suppression 152
Ovum see Oocyte
Oxygen
 ductus arteriosus 104
 placental transport 76–9
Oxytocin 170–71
 control of release 171
  lactation 141, 144–5, 146
  oestrogens and 169
  parturition 137, 146
 effects 170
  fetus ejection reflex 137,
   146
  milk ejection reflex 21,
   144–5, 146
  parturition 137
  placental separation 152
  post partum 152
  prostaglandin release
   135, 176
  sperm transport 64
  uterine haemorrhage 152
 neonatal 123
 receptors 168

Pacemaker potentials,
  myometrial 132
Pancreas 123–4
Paradoxical sleep 127–8
Paramesonephric (Müllerian)
  ducts 6–10
Parathyroid hormone (PTH)
  124
Parity 99
Parturition 130–37
 ACTH release 119
 behaviour during and after
  154–5
 breast sensitivity after 141
 cervix and 133
 definition 130
 environment for 137, 154
 fear of 137

fetal physiology during
131-2
maternal physiology during
131
myometrium and 132,
133-5, 145
nycthemeral rhythmicity 137
oestrogens 132, 135, 136
onset of 130, 133-4
oxytocin 135, 137
progesterone 84, 132, 133-4,
135, 172
prostaglandins 135-6
puerperium 141
stages of 130-31
timing of onset 20
human 136-7
sheep 136
Parvicellular neurosecretory
system 24
Penis
at twelve 8-9
development 7-10
ejaculation 50, 61, 63
erection 61
growth at puberty 14, 160
oestrogens and 61
sensitivity 61
sexual response 63
structure 50
Perivitelline space 66
Pethidine 128
Peyer's patches 90, 141
PG *see* Prostaglandins
Phenylethanolamine-N-methyl
transferase (PNMT) 122,
123
Pheromones
behaviour 20, 46, 47
puberty 17
Phosphatidylglycerol 106
Phospholipase 135
Phospholipids 81, 125, 135
Phosphorus 81
Phosphorylase 126
Pineal gland 24-5, 162
puberty 17, 20, 25
seasonal breeding 19, 163
Pituitary gland
anterior
activation at puberty
14-17
binding of oestrogens 27
control 19, 22-7
development 116
fetal 116-17, 118-19
FSH and LH 39, 57-8
GnRH, effect of 14-17,
39-43, 58, 163
lactogenesis, role in 143
parturition and 136
pregnancy 85
prolactin 85, 173
posterior 22, 64
Placenta, placental 73-83
amniotic fluid, exchange
with 112
barrier 73, 75-6
blood flow 74-5, 79, 100
degeneration 99
delivery of 131
discoid 73
enzymes 119-22, 136
fetal growth 99

feto-placental unit 119-22,
136
formation 70, 73
growth 97-8
haemo-chorial 70, 73, 90
haemodialysis 111
hormones 73, 76, 82, 83-4,
164-5
immunological role 73
ischaemia 101
lactogenesis, role in 143
local block of myometrium
134
oestrogen synthesis 119-22,
136, 170
oxygen utilization 76
parturition, role in 136
potential difference 80
prostaglandin synthesis 135
structure 73-4
transfusion 104-5
transport 73, 75-82
ACTH 119
albumins 81
amino acids 80, 81
antipyrine 75
barbiturates 82
bilirubin 109-10
bilirubin glucuronide
109
calcium 80, 81, 124
carbon dioxide 76, 77,
79, 82
chloride 75, 81
cholesterol 81
cortisol 119-22
creatinine 81, 82
cystine 80
drugs 82, 128
electrolytes 80
fatty acids 81, 125
glucose 80, 81
hormones 81, 116
human growth hormone
116
immunoglobulins 81,
92-3, 94
iodide 80
iron 80, 81
ketone bodies 125
lactic acid 88
magnesium 81
oestrogens 81-2
opiates 82
oxygen 76-9
phospholipids 125
phosphorus 81
potassium 80, 81
progesterone 81
prolactin 116
protein 80-81
sodium 75, 81
streptomycin 82
sulphonamides 82
testosterone 81-2
thyroxine 81, 118
triglycerides 125
urea 75, 81, 82
uric acid 81, 82
vitamins 81, 82
vitamin D and deriva-
tives 124
water 75
villi 73-5, 80, 85, 92

Plasma cells 90, 91
Plasma protein 86
Plasma volume, maternal
during pregnancy 86
Pneumococci 94
PNMT *see* Phenylethanolamine-
N-methyl transferase
Polar bodies 33, 37, 67
Polycystic ovary syndrome 162,
166
Polyhydramnios 114, 136
Polyspermy, block to 37, 66-7
Potter's syndrome 111, 114
Pre-eclampsia 87
Pregnancy 73-95
behavioural changes 89
cervix changes 130
corpus luteum 38-40
duration 96, 122, 136-7
ectopic 167
fat storage during 88-9, 152
fluid retention during 88
hormone levels during 84
immunology of 89-94
immunoglobulin levels
during 92
initiation 40, 72, 83
mammary gland changes
141-2
maternal physiology during
83-9
cardiovascular 86-7
endocrinology 83-6
gastrointestinal 88
metabolic 87
renal 87
respiratory 87
oestrogens, effect of during
169
pelvic tissue changes 130
skin changes 87
twin 75, 86, 99, 165
vaginal changes 130
weight change 88-9
Pregnanediol 110, 114, 172-3
Pregnenolone 119-21, 157, 171
Premature babies
bilirubin metabolism 110
hypertyrosinaemia 111
hyponatraemia 112
immunoglobulins 93
jaundice 110
sodium retention 112
Premenstrual tension (PMT) 46
Primary sex cords 4-5
Primate, brain differentiation 11
Primordial germ cells 4-5, 32-3
PRL *see* Prolactin
Progestagens 171-3
cervix 64
chemical characteristics 157,
171
effects 171-2
bilirubin conjugation,
suppression of 110
contraceptive 64
masculinizing 10, 12
oviduct 45
stimulation of LH
release 42
uterus 44-5
vagina 20
induced hermaphroditism 3,
10

levels 159
  menstrual cycle 41
  luteal 38
menstrual cycle 38–42
receptors 44–5
sites of synthesis 171
see also Progesterone
Progesterone 171–73
  amniotic fluid 114
  binding 27, 134, 172
  biosynthesis 121, 157
  chemical formula 121, 157
  effects 171–72
    anaesthetic 172
    behavioural 172
    body temperature 41,
      46, 172
    breast development 140
      141, 172
    cervix, uterine 64, 172
    endometrium 44–5,
      71–2, 73, 172
    feedback 172
    lactogenesis 85, 142–4
      148, 172
    maternal behaviour 172
    metabolic 87
    myometrium 45, 132–4
    oviduct 45, 172
    oxytocin release 172
    prolactin release 142–4
    prostaglandin synthesis
      135, 176
    sodium and water reten-
      tion 172
    uterine blood flow 75
    uterine growth 89
    vagina 20, 46
  feto-placental unit and 119,
    121, 172
  levels 159
    menstrual cycle 41
    pregnant mother 84,
      133–4
    luteal 38–39
  menstrual cycle 37–42
  placental transport 81–82
  receptors 44–5, 169
  stimulation of LH release 42
  withdrawal, and onset of
    labour 133–4
Prolactin 173–4
  amniotic fluid 114, 116
  control of release 174
    bromocriptine 144
    coitus-induced 21
    dopamine 174–5
    oestrogens 142–4, 169
    olfactory stimuli 144
    progesterone 142–4
    suckling 21, 144
    thyrotrophin-releasing
      hormone (TRH)
      174, 175
  effects 173
    breast growth 140
    corticotrophic in fetus
      118
    lactogenic 85, 140,
      142–4, 148
    luteotrophic 83
    ovarian inhibition 173
  levels 158
    amniotic fluid 116
    fetal 116–17

neonatal 117
  pregnant mother 84, 85,
    142
  puberty 16
  synthesis in pituitary 173
Prolactin release inhibiting
  hormone 174–5
Prostacyclins 104, 135
Prostaglandin synthetase 135
Prostaglandins (PG and
  PGF2α) 175–6
  control of release 135, 176
  effects 175–6
    cervix, uterine 133
    ductus arteriosus 104
    implantation 70
    luteolysis 38–9, 71, 83,
      175
    oxytocic 175
    parturition 135, 175
    sperm transport 64,
      175–6
  oestrogens and 135, 168
  synthesis 135, 175
Prostate 7–8, 50, 60, 61, 160
Protein
  fetal accumulation of 96
  placental transfer of 80–81
PTH *see* Parathyroid hormone
Puberty 12–18
  adrenarche 17–18
  amygdala, role of 17
  breast development 14, 140
  central nervous system, and
    17
  critical body weight theory
    17
  genitalia development 12–14
  GnRH, role in 14–17, 164
  gonadostat theory 16–17
  growth during 13–14
  hair development 9, 13–14
  hormonal changes 14–18,
    48, 158–9
  light, effect of 12, 17, 20, 25
  nutrition, effect of 12
  ovarian changes 32–3
  physical changes 13–14
  pineal, role of 17, 20, 25
  precocious 17, 20, 25, 167
  psychological changes 14
  testicular changes 14, 52
Puerperium 141
Pulmonary circulation, fetal
  101, 103

Rabbit 21, 43, 80, 116, 125,
  133–4, 164
Rat
  brain sexual differentiation
    10–11, 160
  brown adipose tissue 125
  fat deposition in pregnancy
    88–9
  fetal growth 100–101, 116
  glucagon 124
  ketone utilization 125
  oestrous cycles 10–11, 19,
    43, 166–7
  prolactin
    luteotrophic function 83,
      173
    release by coitus 21, 173
5α-Reductase 160
  genetic deficiency 8–9

in epididymis 58
Reflex ovulation, *see* Ovulation,
  reflex
Rejection, immune 89–90
Relaxin 133, 176
Renal blood flow 86, 111
Renal function
  fetus and neonate 111–12,
    113–14
  pregnant mother 87
Renin 46, 75, 169
Reserpine 173
Respiratory distress syndrome,
  idiopathic (IRDS) 106,
  122
Respiratory system
  fetus and neonate 106–8
  pregnant mother 87
Rete cords 5
Rete testis 51, 57
Retinohypothalamic projection
  24–5
Reverse tri-iodothyronine (rT3)
  118
RER *see* Rough endoplasmic
  reticulum
Ribonucleic acid (RNA) 67,
  142, 160
RNA *see* Ribonucleic acid
Rotaviruses 150

Scrotum 7, 9, 50–51, 63
Seasonal breeding 19
Secondary sex cords 4–5
Semen 60, 63
  see also Spermatozoa
Seminal fluid 60
Seminal vesicles 7–8, 50, 60,
  160
Seminiferous tubules 51–7
  tubular fluid 57
Sertoli cells 52, 55–8
Serum IgA 91
Sex
  cords, primary and
    secondary 4
  genetic determination 1–5
  gonadal dimorphism 4–5, 7
Sex-hormone binding globulin
  (SHBG) 117, 161
Sexual behaviour
  changes at puberty 14
  description 61–4
  differentiation 10–12, 160
  effect of hormones 10–12,
    43, 61–2
  menstrual cycle 46–7
  oestrogens and 169
  oestrus 29
  olfactory stimuli 20, 47, 62
  tactile stimuli 62
  visual stimuli 20, 62
Sexual differentiation 1–14
  abnormal 3, 8–10
  androgens and 6–12, 117
  brain, and 10–12, 160, 169
  genetics of 1–4
  genitalia, of 6–10
  gonadal 4–6
  puberty at 10–12
Sexual intercourse/response
  62–3
Sexually dimorphic nucleus 11
Sexually transmissible diseases
  64

Sheehan's syndrome 174
Sheep
  cortisol, and parturition 136
  fetus
    ACTH infusion 136
    adrenal cortex 136, 173
    adrenalectomy 136
    amniotic fluid 113
    chemoreceptors 107-8
    circulation 101-3
    corticosteroids 106, 122, 173
    growth 100, 116
    hypophysectomy 116, 136
    lung surfactant 106
    pituitary gland 116, 118-19, 136
    renal blood flow 111
    sympathetic activation 107
    urine flow 113
  immunity, transfer of 93
  luteolysis 38-9
  neonatal breathing 107-8
  nutrition 100
  parturition 122, 136, 137
  placenta 75, 76-7, 173
  seasonal breeding 19
Skin, fetal 112
Sleep
  LH levels 20
  neonatal 127-8
  prolactin 175
  rapid-eye-movement (REM) 127-8
Small-for-dates (SFD) babies 94, 96, 100
Smell, *see* Olfactory
Smoking 100, 106
Sodium
  placental transport 75, 80, 81
  pump in mammary secretory cell 148
Somatotrophin 116
Sound 21
Sparteine 170
Spermatids 53-6
Spermatocyte 53-4, 57
Spermatogenesis
  cyclical nature 56-7
  description 53-7
  endocrine control 57-8, 160
  location 52
  temperature, and 51
Spermatogonia 4-5, 52-7
Spermatozoa
  acrosome reaction 65-6
  activation 65-6
  antigens 90
  capacitation 64-5
  definition 1
  development 51-60
  emission 63
  lifespan 64
  maturation 51, 160, 161
  motility 57, 60, 65, 66
  oocyte fusion and penetration 33
  receptors 65
  remodelling (spermiogenesis) 53-6
  storage 51
  structure 59

transport in female tract 64-5
transport in male tract 51, 57-60, 63
see also Semen
Spermiogenesis (spermeteliosis) 53-6
Spina bifida 114
Spinnbarkeit 64, 172
Spleen 91, 92
Staphylococci 94
Steroidogenic pathways
  in developing follicular cells 35-6
Stigma, of the follicle 37
Stress 21-2, 43, 137, 144-5, 159, 164, 171, 174
Suckling
  depression of 128
  effects
    gonadotrophin inhibition 21, 43, 139, 152, 164
    milk ejection 144-6
    milk removal 144, 145
    oxytocin release 144-6, 152
    pleasure 139, 152
    prolactin release 21, 143, 144, 174
Supine hypotension syndrome 86
Suprachiasmatic nucleus 19, 43
Surfactant 106, 114, 118, 125
Surge, LH 10-11, 37, 40-43
Syncytiotrophoblast
  formation 69, 70, 73
  immunological role 90, 92
  in mature placenta 74
  source of hCG 164
  source of hPL 85, 165
Syngamy 67

T cells *see* Thymus-derived lymphocytes
T4 *see* Thyroxine
Tactile stimuli 21
Tanycytes, ependymal 24-5, 163
Temperature
  menstrual cycle 41, 172
  testis 51
Testicular feminization syndrome 3, 9
Testis
  androgens from 52-3, 57-8
  blood supply 51
  blood-testis barrier 52
  compartments 52
  cords 5
  descent 50-51
  development 4-7, 50-52
  endocrine function 52-3, 57, 58
  fetal 6-8, 50-52, 117
  interstitial (Leydig) cell 6-7, 52-3, 57-8, 117, 160
  migration 50-51
  puberty 14, 52
  regression 61
  structure 50-51
  temperature 51
Testosterone 157-162
  aromatization to oestradiol 11, 27, 160

binding in brain 27
binding protein 53, 160
biosynthesis 52, 157, 160
conversion to DHT 7-9, 58-9, 160
effects 160-61
  behaviour 61
  masculinizing 6-8
  sperm maturation 58-9
  spermatogenesis 57
levels 158
  castration 61
  fetus 6, 117
  menstrual cycle 41
  neonatal 10-11, 52
placental transport 81-82
receptors 58
stimuli to release 22, 57-8, 161
synthesis 35-6, 52-3
see also Androgens
Theca interna and externa 32-6
Thymus-derived lymphocytes (T cells) 90
Thyrocalcitonin (TCT) 124
Thyroid gland 99, 118
Thyroid stimulating hormone (TSH) 118
Thyrotrophin releasing hormone (TRH) 116, 174, 175
Thyroxine (T4)
  breast growth 140
  fetal 118
  neonatal metabolism 127
  placental transfer 81
T lymphocytes 90
Touch 21
Transferrin 80
Tri-iodothyronine 118
  see also Reverse tri-iodothyronine
Trophoblast (trophectoderm) 67, 69, 70, 73-4, 75, 83, 90, 136, 164
Tunica albuginea 4-5
Turner's syndrome 2-5
Twin pregnancy 75, 86, 99, 136
Tyrosine 111

Umbilical arteries 101, 122
Umbilical cord
  amniotic fluid, exchange with 112
  clamping 105, 110, 151
  compression during labour 131-2
Umbilical vein 101
Urea 81, 82, 111, 112, 114, 115
Ureter 7-8
Urethra 7-8, 50
Urethral folds 7, 9
Uric acid 81, 82, 115
Urogenital sinus 7-8
Uterus, uterine
  blood flow, 75, 76, 89, 100, 101, 133, 168
  cervix *see* Cervix, uterine
  contractions 45, 63, 130-33, 152
  development 7-8
  endometrium 30, 39, 44-5, 69-72, 73, 135, 168, 170, 172
  enlargement in pregnancy 89

glands 44–5, 69, 70, 71, 73
haemorrhage 152
hysterectomy 83
inertia 137
ligaments 130–31
luteolysis, role in 38–9, 83
menopause and 47
menstrual cycle 44–5
milk 70
myometrium 30, 44–5, 69, 74, 122, 132–4, 135, 145, 152, 168, 172
oestrogens, effects of 44–5, 71–2, 89, 132–3, 135, 136, 168, 170
oxytocin 135, 137, 152
parturition 130–37
postpartum 152
progesterone, effects of 45, 71–2, 73, 89, 132–4, 135, 172
prolapse 131
prostaglandins and 135–7
sperm transport 64–5

stretch 135, 137
structure 29–30

Vagina, vaginal
development 7–8
menopause 47–8, 170
menstrual cycle 46
oestrogens, effect of 20, 46, 168
pregnancy, changes during 130
puberty, changes at 14
secretions, and sexual behaviour 20, 46
sexual response 63
sperm transport 64
structure 30
Vas deferens 7–8, 50–51, 57–60, 160
Vasopressin 123
Vasotocin 123
Venereal diseases 64
Veratrum californicum 136
Villi, placental 73–5, 80, 85, 92
Visual stimuli 20

Vitamin C 111
Vitamin D and derivatives 124, 151
Vitamins 81, 82, 150, 151
Vitelline membrane 66
Vomiting 89

Water
fetal 97
placental transport 75, 79
retention in pregnancy 88
Weaning 153
Weight change in pregnancy, 86, 88–9
Whey 149
Whitten effect 20

X-chromosome 1–5

Y-chromosome 1–5, 7, 9, 50
Yolk sac 4, 32, 69

Zona
pellucida 32, 34, 65–6, 71
reaction 65, 67